Praise for *Ashes Transformed*

What would be a religiously faithful response to the terror of September 11? Here are dozens of them gathered in this wise, courageous, hopeful book by respected and beloved therapist and Christian healer Tilda Norberg. This moving collection of stories—profound, mysterious, and heart-wrenching—offers new images of healing and hope in the aftermath of September 11 and widens out to reach the trauma, pain, and evil that can beset any life. Savoring and praying over these stories will reawaken one's awe at the simplicity and surprise of God's love.

ROBERT D. WEBBER
Professor of New Testament Emeritus
Lancaster Theological Seminary
Lancaster, Pennsylvania

In *Ashes Transformed* the universal experiences of trauma, grief, and healing are shared by many voices out of the World Trade Center tragedy. The book invites the reader to contemplate slowly, one story at a time. Tilda Norberg's therapeutic skills and spiritual depth shine through the prayer suggestions that follow each story. She invites the reader to reflect upon his or her own experiences of struggle or pain and to lift them up to God. This is more than a book—it is a transforming experience.

GWEN AND DALE WHITE
GWEN—Spiritual life retreat and workshop leader
DALE—Bishop, The United Methodist Church
Newport, Rhode Island

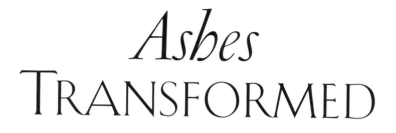

Ashes
Transformed

Healing from Trauma

43 Stories of Faith

TILDA NORBERG

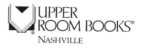

UPPER
ROOM BOOKS®
NASHVILLE

The publisher gratefully acknowledges permission to reprint the following copyrighted material:
Anne Mimi Sammis for permission to use photographs of her sculptures:
Peace Is Here, Visitation, 9/11, Rainbow of Souls, Embrace of Life II (also used on cover), *He Has the Whole World in His Hands, Forgiveness, Dove of Peace.*
Photographs on pages 24, 40, 72, 78, 112, 148, 156, 174, and 186 by Beau Jones/IDC.

Excerpt from "A Service of Word and Table I." Copyright © 1979, 1980, 1985, 1989 The United Methodist Publishing House. Used by permission.

Cover and Interior Design: Bruce Gore/Gore Studio, Inc.
Cover Photo: Beau Jones/Images Design Company
Author Photo: Susan Stevenson, Staten Island
Interior Icon Development: Jim Osborn
First Printing: 2002

Library of Congress Cataloging-in-Publication Data
Norberg, Tilda.
Ashes transformed : healing from trauma / Tilda Norberg.
    p.   cm.
ISBN 0-8358-0986-2
1. Spiritual healing. 2. Prayer—Christianity. 3. September 11 Terrorist Attacks, 2001—Religious aspects—Christianity. I. Title.
BV227 .N665 2003
248.8'6—dc21   2002013292
Printed in the United States of America

TO ALL WHO TOLD THEIR STORIES

and

TO GEORGE McCLAIN,
most loving of husbands,
who holds my hand.

SPECIAL THANKS TO
Bette Sohm, whose cheerful help is a gift;
Everett Wabst, who has eyes of faith;
Wanda Craner, Rhoda Glick, and Sara Goold,
partners in Gestalt Pastoral Care Ecumenical Associates, who said,
"Why not you?"
and William Rickard,
who knew that healing was possible.

CONTENTS

All of the stories in this book are true. Where first and last names are used, they are the actual name of the individual telling the story. Stories told in the first person are my own experiences.

A few persons requested that their names not be used to protect their privacy. In these instances, I created a fictional first name and relocated the context to another geographic area. In all other respects I wrote the stories just as they were told to me.

Healing from Trauma

WE ARE A world of terrorized and traumatized people. Most Americans had front-row seats to the tragic events of September 11, 2001, as again and again the television networks showed the crashing planes and burning, collapsing buildings. We felt as if we personally and directly experienced the disaster. Even people thousands of miles physically from the crash sites were there emotionally and spiritually.

The horrific images seared into our minds and hearts, firmly implanting traumatic reactions. Many people had nightmares, flashbacks, panic attacks, and bodies ready for fight or flight. Others became numb, not ready to feel anything, trying hard to return to the way things were on September 10. Still others felt that the world irrevocably tilted—never again could we return to our former sense of innocence and trust that the world is generally safe. No longer would we be able simply to board a plane and fly without knotted muscles and sweaty palms. Never again could we trust people we don't know. Never again would we be free of fear and anxiety, and healing seemed a mere fantasy. Fresh trauma typically engenders such reactions.

In addition to this shared national trauma, many persons battle private histories of other devastating events.

Nightmarish memories of childhood sexual abuse, of rape or other violence, of accidents or the mayhem of earthquakes and tornadoes can haunt us for a lifetime. So can parents' verbal cruelty that crushes the spirit of children, or schools that teach students to regard themselves as stupid, or demeaning work situations that demand rigid conformity and dronelike activity. Racism, sexism, classism, and homophobia can wound deeply too, for prejudice erodes the very personhood of its targets. Years of experience as a psychotherapist convince me that large numbers of us carry painful, often frightening wounds that drag us down and sap our physical energy, emotional resilience, and spiritual joy.

TYPICAL RESPONSES TO TRAUMA

When newly traumatized, we tumble about in an ocean of reactions. Although we may feel agonizingly out of control, trauma produces some fairly predictable responses.

First, *a traumatic event produces an emotional and spiritual storm.* As the events of September 11 unfolded, they produced an intense welter of red-hot emotions and spiritual anguish. People reported feeling terrified, enraged, panicked, nauseated, deserted by God, and in despair. They felt as if the ground under them had collapsed and they were falling into a pit of uncertainty and fear.

Second, when people directly experience a terrible event, *they file away images and stories of the event in their memory.* Typically trauma engages our need to know what happened. So in addition to scenes we may have witnessed, we create images of scenes we could not have witnessed. Since 9/11 many people carry images and stories their imaginations have created, depicting, for example, what those final minutes must have been like for the passengers on the four planes or what happened to people in the towers at the moment the floors gave way. In an effort to heal, we may mentally replay the "movie" again and again. Later flashbacks may also focus on these "movies."

The third cluster of reactions involves *denial and paralysis*. On September 11 we couldn't quite grasp the reality of this horror, no matter how many newscasts we watched. "I just can't believe it" was the topic of conversation around the country. The words *surreal* and *unthinkable* entered our national vocabulary in a new way. Emotions were so intense that they felt too big to express. Like deer caught in headlights, people were stunned into paralysis, as if body and spirit were too small to embrace the reactions inside.

Paralysis is not necessarily bad. It does not reveal cowardice, emotional weakness, or spiritual failure. Numbness is actually a wonderful way to protect ourselves from emotions for which we are not ready. Out of numbness can emerge a sort of inner organization in which it is possible to feel one emotion at a time instead of all of them at once. Numbness can preserve us until we find the right time and place to let go. Thank God we can create emotional fire walls that keep us from being consumed with pain or fear.

At this stage people speak of fatigue, nausea, and blankness. Some feel depressed and withdrawn, wanting only to sleep. Conversely, others report nightmares and sleeping difficulties. Still others find they cannot pray. At this point persons are highly vulnerable to alcohol and drug abuse.

Anything that might take away the intense emotions can seem like a life raft.

Fourth, *memories and emotions that are not expressed in depth find a home in the body's muscles.* Although numbing one's awareness of emotional and spiritual distress is possible, the distress has not gone away. Instead it has become physically embodied in tense and achy muscles, sore and stiff joints, constricted breathing, increased heart rate, or a stomach full of knots. Sometimes the embodiment of childhood memories is so complete that the trauma is "forgotten," lost to awareness. But inside our muscles is a carefully guarded time capsule full of emotions and memories almost fresh in intensity. It is as if we grow an emotional and spiritual cyst around the pain.

The beauty of embodied memories is that for the time being we don't feel so assaulted and devastated. The catch is that we may find it difficult to feel any emotion at all with intensity and passion, and we may still have physical reactions such as headaches, backaches, shoulder pain, and disrupted digestion or sleep.

At this stage familiar routines comfort us. Going through the motions, doing ordinary things, can make life seem almost normal again. Although we may regain an uneasy calm, real healing has not occurred; and we may get stuck in this stage. Repetitious routines may act like a drug, and we may plod along for years, half alive and numb to the anguish seething below the surface.

When trauma lasts for years, as often is true with childhood physical or sexual abuse, new traumatic experiences typically get directed to one or more interior time capsules.

Such setting aside is a coping technique that enables a young child to survive truly unbearable experiences.

Helps for Genuine Healing: Therapy and Prayer

Genuine healing from trauma involves every part of us: body, emotions, and spirit. Opening the cyst of emotions and memories requires willingness to revisit the trauma as many times as needed. Allowing ourselves to go back and relive what previously was too frightening and overwhelming is hard work. However, we can take it in small doses; the cyst can drain slowly. The trauma needn't overwhelm us again. We can go back in time and experience some of our feelings and physical reactions and return to the present when we want.

Because healing from trauma involves a complex and sometimes frightening process, most people need the assistance of a good therapist. For persons of faith, finding a therapist who at least respects their Christian commitment is important, even if that is not a shared commitment. When emotional and physical release can occur in the context of recognizing God's faithful, healing presence, the process tends to be much easier and faster. For this reason a spiritual director can greatly enhance the healing process as well.

The knowledge that your loving God is with you can enable you to face the monsters inside. The belief that Jesus has overcome death and evil equips you to look at death and evil in the face. Willingness to invite Jesus to accompany you to the scene of your living nightmare can open the door to marvelous healing that enlarges and reframes old memories to include the presence of the Lord. Healing grace can empower you to forgive and to shape your life as an advocate for others in misery.

I know that painful experiences, no matter how catastrophic, can be healed through a combination of inner work and prayer. You do not forget the experiences, of course, but they no longer have the power to terrify you and control your reactions. Whatever your age, talents, history, or handicaps, God works to bring you to the particular wholeness God wills for you. I know this truth from many years in healing ministry and as a Gestalt Pastoral psychotherapist. I know it best, however, as a result of my own healing from a terrible trauma.

My Story

My story reaches back to my junior year in high school in 1959 when I was sixteen years old. On Easter Sunday that year, a plane crashed just short of the airport runway in Saginaw, Michigan. My mother and father were among the forty-seven passengers who were killed instantly. I was at the airport waiting to pick them up and witnessed the accident.

The plane exploded into a tremendous roaring fireball that ripped apart the fabric of my life. I knew immediately that my parents were dead; no one could possibly have survived that inferno.

The fire burned fiercely through the night as pockets of fuel continued to ignite, engulfing and devouring the plane, reducing it to a heap of twisted metal in a muddy cornfield. Rescue workers were helpless in the face of the intense heat and smoke.

Inside the airport was pandemonium. Sirens wailed; alarms clanged; red lights flashed. People screamed hysterically, fainted, clutched one another. Panicked staff ran about in shock. I was sick to my stomach, my heart beating wildly, my throat constricted, my legs like jelly. A scream rose in my throat, but I fought it back. I was terrified and shaking but determined not to lose control or get hysterical.

Suddenly it seemed as if a screen was pulled down over the airport interior, and all I saw was a vivid, slightly sparkly whiteness, something like a movie screen on which images are projected. The cacophony of sounds disappeared as well, and in its place came a deep silence. I was not in a trance, however; I remained aware of the burning plane outside and of my own intense physical reactions.

Then I saw Jesus. He stood directly in front of me and gazed at me with great love. I don't mean I saw him with my mind's eye, as I have many times since. I saw him with physical eyes, perceiving him in the same way I see my dog curled up at my feet. His clothing glowed, and I knew that I was seeing his resurrected body. Jesus spoke to me, and I heard seven words with physical ears: "Don't be afraid; I'm always with you." He repeated these words many times, as if to make sure that I understood and would be certain for the rest of my life that he had indeed spoken to me. I have no idea whether the encounter took a few minutes or much longer, but I do know that for some time I stood in wordless ecstasy with Jesus.

After a time I could no longer see him, and the screaming chaos of the Saginaw airport roared back into focus. I was still terrified and nauseous as the burning plane seared its way into the front of my consciousness again. At the very same time I felt profoundly rooted in God's love for me and my parents. I was like a tree in a hurricane, bent over and stripped of leaves and branches but deeply anchored in soil that would not let me go. At that moment I knew in my bones that my life would not be trouble free, but I also knew that Jesus would be there. I knew that my parents were with him and that eventually I would be all right. I also sensed in a sixteen-year-old way that I could not let my encounter with Jesus become a magic tranquilizer that would keep me from feeling pain and grief. Clearly, I was still in profound shock as a severely traumatized, newly orphaned teenager. I would have to go through the experience, but I could hold onto the promise that Jesus would be with me.

Right away I began to learn what it means to endure a terrible experience but to do so with Jesus there. As soon as the vision of the risen Jesus faded, I began hearing the Easter anthem we had sung that morning in church. I heard this music not with physical ears but in my "mind's ear." Like a tape playing over and over, the music stayed with me constantly for the next three weeks. I heard it as my parents' bodies were identified, and as my sister and I picked out their caskets. I heard it at the funeral. I heard it as I watched horrifying images of the crash on television and as I tried to concentrate in school. I heard it when most of my friends avoided me because they just couldn't figure out what to say.

As the Easter anthem captured my attention again and again, I began to understand what Jesus meant when he said he would always be with me. I most certainly went through a devastating time but was constantly reminded that this music proclaiming God's victory over death was just as real as the plane crash. Holding these two experiences together brought me tremendous healing.

Even after experiencing the marvelous vision of Jesus in the airport and the music afterward, in the following years I still had plenty of difficult inner work to do. I physically ached for my parents and my old, secure life. I saw the potential for disaster everywhere, everyday. My body jumped at loud noises. The sound of a plane flying low made me want to run and cover my ears. I avoided the Saginaw airport until I drove out there alone one day, naively hoping to conquer my fear. I shook violently as I watched a few planes land and finally left after I threw up beside the chain-link fence.

Even though the vision of Jesus at the airport was my center and offered a place of profound healing and rest, my body still carried reactions to the disaster. I wondered how I could feel so fearful when Jesus himself told me not to be afraid. I didn't realize that I was suffering from post-traumatic stress disorder; back then no one even had a name for this condition.

Slowly I came to understand that Jesus' words to me did not call me to pretend that I was just fine, but instead they invited me to work on my fear until it was gone. I entered therapy and worked hard until I could assimilate the healing Jesus had offered. Quite soon I became strong enough to reexperience the crash, to scream the screams I had stifled in the airport, and to face head-on the imaginary movie I had created of my parents' last moments. My healing process was wrenching, but Jesus' presence made it infinitely easier. I did not have to reenter those feelings alone; he went with me. Each time I took the journey back in time to the terror and ecstasy of that Easter Sunday, I returned to the present time feeling lighter. My pain was being healed, and I was maturing.

My pastor, William "Tex" Rickard of State Street Methodist Church in Saginaw, spent a great deal of time with me, helping me understand that God did not cause the plane to fall out of the sky, nor did God allow the crash in order to teach me or anyone else a lesson. The crash was neither punishment nor evidence that God didn't care. Rather, when the disaster happened (because of a defective design in the plane's deicing mechanism) God set out immediately to redeem it.

For the next several years Tex and his wife, Mary, embodied the love of God for my sister and me. A few months after the crash they invited us to live with them, and we stayed with them until we both finished college.

Now I know that this marvelous encounter with the risen Christ at the Saginaw airport, together with the subsequent healing process, planted the seeds of my call to ordained ministry. It also undergirded my later decision to train as a psychotherapist and was crucial in my discovery of a new integration of healing ministry with Gestalt psychotherapy, which I named Gestalt Pastoral Care. When working with other trauma survivors I bring personal experience that makes me certain that terrible traumas can be healed through hard work and prayer for healing. Although as a therapist I seldom speak about my own experience, I know the territory of trauma from the inside; this knowledge greatly helps people in their own difficult healing process.

The more healing I undergo, the more I understand one of the most magnificent truths of the Christian faith: *God can turn our worst pain into the source of our giftedness.* It is no accident that my life's work involves helping people invite Jesus into the worst moments of their lives.

When the planes hit the World Trade towers and the Pentagon and crashed in that Pennsylvania field, I was, of course, stunned and horrified, but I also had an odd sense of déjà vu. Although the devastation of 9/11 occurred on a much larger scale than my teenage trauma, it still felt familiar. I felt I knew something of the contours of what the nation was feeling, and I sensed that I had already worked through many issues now facing the American people.

I was amazed to discover that the attacks did not trigger my old trauma; instead they reaffirmed the depth of my healing over the years. I also felt an immediate passion for collecting the stories of others who experienced God's healing presence in connection with the 9/11 disaster.

OUR STORIES AFTER SEPTEMBER 11

I did not have to search far for stories of faith related to September 11. I heard them in the natural course of talking with my friends, family, students, and colleagues about what had happened to them since then. Because I live on Staten Island, I could talk to people directly involved in the disaster. Many of my neighbors make the thirty-minute daily commute on the Staten Island ferry to the lower tip of Manhattan. From the ferry terminal it is just a short walk to the World Trade towers site and Wall Street. The financial district feels like part of our neighborhood.

Staten Islanders were hit hard on September 11. Many ran in terror for their lives, and most folks on Staten Island know at least one person who perished. Although Staten Island has by far the smallest population of New York City's five boroughs, we lost more firefighters and police officers than any other borough.

As friends and neighbors shared their stories, they also suggested other people to contact. A simple phone call to a stranger usually produced another moving story of God's healing presence, active and evident in the aftermath of the horrific events. News of magnificent ministry responses to the tragedy traveled on the church grapevine. Many churches flung open their doors on September 11 and have continued to find creative ways of caring for their communities.

Soon I became convinced that God has been extraordinarily active in the lives of ordinary people since the tragedy. On the day of the attacks, God already was beginning the process of healing. With eyes of faith many persons have been able to see signs of God's merciful love even in the midst of their fear and sorrow. Though confronted with stark evil, they have been comforted, challenged, and astonished by evidence of God's faithful presence. They have been empowered to let go of terrifying emotions. Many people of faith have been spurred to affirm a new global perspective that advocates sharing the world's resources with all people. Some have been moved to stop chasing material possessions, hearing again a still small voice saying, "You shall have no other gods before me" (Exod. 20:3).

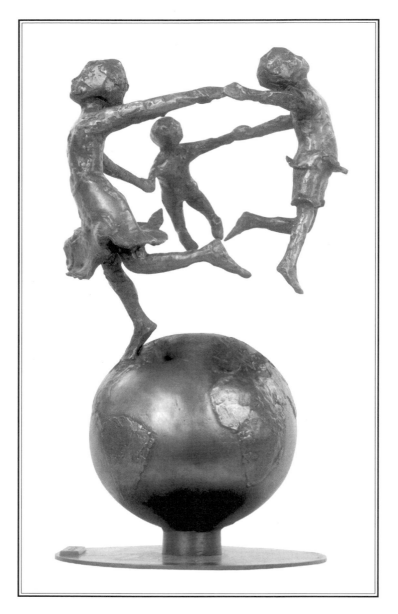

PEACE IS HERE

Healing through Faith Imagination

⌒

THE FOLLOWING collection of stories of God's mercy and healing hints at the myriad ways God was at work just after the attack. Although these stories refer to 9/11 and are personal and specific to a particular person or group, they are not essentially private, nor do they apply only to this national trauma. I believe that the church can allow these experiences and responses of faith to heal many different wounds. No matter what pain we carry, God can speak to us personally through these stories. Perhaps they can also call us to repentance, both public and private, and spur us to action. These small stories help make up The Story, the great narrative of God's love and mercy through the ages. In that sense they are gospel, which means "good news."

NO EASY ANSWERS

By recording these stories I do not intend to suggest that one or two experiences of God's healing, no matter how wondrous or life-changing, can instantly accomplish complete healing. Each of these stories is like a single pearl on a long string; more healing stories will emerge from each life. Even when God intervenes mightily, such as melting a tumor within minutes or pouring miraculous spiritual comfort on breathtaking pain, healing remains a process that continues as long as you remain open to God's presence. You can expect an awareness of God's presence to break into your life many times as God continually invites you to take yet another step toward wholeness.

No easy answers, magic therapies, or prayer techniques can simply erase the immense impact of trauma. Genuine healing from trauma never involves ignoring its enormity or "stuffing" the flow of emotions that naturally result. Nor can facile or even well-reasoned explanations adequately address heartfelt, anguished questions. Quoting Bible verses, even verses that glow with faith and hope, in an attempt to erase raging emotions and spiritual desolation may only make matters worse. Hearing sermons that urge us to trust in God's love during a time of trauma may wind up making some people even angrier at God.

Sometimes you are in so much pain that you cannot pray. When you try, your prayer seems to fall with a thud to the floor, and when you try to open yourself to God's presence, you encounter a whole lot of nothing. God seems to have vanished, and all you have left are emotions and spirit tangled with pain, anger, and desolation. The truth is that when you have experienced trauma, you cannot always muster the faith to claim God's promises for yourself, and you must depend on other people to pray for you. With good reason scripture repeatedly urges Jesus' followers to uphold one another in prayer.

At this point grace comes in. Your groping desire for God is enough; God can listen to the prayer you can't yet articulate. God is surely with you in your process of healing, and never more present than when you are in deep pain. God desires your wholeness and willingly meets you in the depths of sorrow, despair, fear, and doubt. God wants to answer your deepest questions, to heal your most wrenching agony, and to reframe your most horrific memories. God wants to replace fear with faith and sorrow with peace that passes understanding but—this is important—not in a way that denies the depth of your feelings. My many years of working with trauma survivors convince me that God does not rob us of our growth process. Instead God accompanies us as we wrestle with our inner turmoil, helping us to work through it until we reach a new place. Truly, the only way around trauma is through it, and God goes through our turmoil with us.

Why?

Sooner or later, when a person of faith undergoes healing from trauma, the question "why?" surfaces. If God is love, why did God allow this terrible thing to happen? Why didn't God stop the terrorists, foil my abuser, arrest the progress of that awful disease, prevent the accident? Even Jesus cried out a tormented "why?" from the cross. "Why?" can be all the more anguished when it seems that God does sometimes intervene. Hundreds of people were supposed to have been in the World Trade towers on 9/11, but for various reasons they weren't, and many praise God for their escape from death.

Knowing that some people escaped the horror does not make it any easier to hold lightly the question of "why?"

Theologians have long tried to figure out why a loving God would allow terrible things to happen. They reason that the gift of free will allows humans the freedom to make disastrous and cruel choices. Or that God created good physical laws to insure that the world is dependable, but these laws sometimes hurt people who inadvertently get in the way. Or that evil exists, and the world is imperfect because of it. Or that evil wins some battles, but the ultimate victory is God's. All of these explanations are true, yet none really answers the "why?" question with finality, and in the end, most conclude that trying to explain why God allows suffering is an impossible task. Humans are simply too limited to fully understand, and the answer lies in the mystery of God's being.

Wanting to know why is natural. *Demanding* to know why can delay healing for years, even decades. Insisting that God or a therapist or a pastor produce an answer that makes sense can be tantamount to staying stuck in the crisis. However, you do not need to ignore such an important question.

I believe God wants to answer your most troubling questions, not with the airtight, logical discourse you may want but in a way that satisfies your heart. Understanding will probably come gradually as you keep the questions open, letting them gently simmer on the back burner. An answer that satisfies *your* heart will not be the same as the one that satisfies someone else. What touches one person deeply may only raise more questions for another. An important part of your healing journey will be to discover your own heart's answer to "why?" When you ask the Holy Spirit to teach you heart answers, that prayer invites healing grace.

Beginning the Journey of Healing

How can you allow this journey to unfold in you? First, you can *surrender to God your idea of how your healing must happen.* When you surrender as best you can, you create space for what God might want to do. The prayer suggestions that accompany the stories offer opportunity to enter into this surrender.

Second, *let yourself express anger at God.* Hanging on to "why?" can be an excellent way to deny your anger and to let your anger fester, perhaps for years. Instead, act like the psalmist—rail at God. Act like a loved child who knows her parents won't reject her when she throws a fit. Give voice to your anger. Write it, paint it, stomp it, yell it. When you finish expressing your anger, ask yourself what happened to "why?" in the process.

Third, you can *reframe your questions to ask "what?" or "how?" instead of "why?"* Something new begins to happen when you ask questions such as:

"What am I experiencing right now?'

"What was God doing when the trauma occurred?"

"What is God doing now?"

"What does Jesus want to tell me?"

"How am I being healed?"

"How is the Holy Spirit inviting me to grow during this time?"

Asking such questions through faith-imagination prayer

has helped countless trauma survivors open themselves to healing grace. (I'll explain faith imagination below.) Furthermore, prayerful exploration of "what?" often gives shape to God's response to your "why?" Answers seem to come gently, surprisingly, almost through the back door. Sometimes it is possible to hold the question "why?" much more loosely because your healing becomes more important than insisting on an answer to the question.

FAITH-IMAGINATION PRAYER

The basis of faith imagination is the belief that God sincerely wants to communicate with you and tries to get through your defenses in order to bring you wholeness. Faith-imagination prayer gives opportunity to delve fully into your feelings while allowing you to open to God's healing.

In faith-imagination prayer you invite God, Jesus, or the Holy Spirit (or another symbol of the Holy One) to work through your imagination so that you can better perceive and cooperate with God's healing work in you. Experience has taught me that God often chooses to work mightily through this simple way of praying. Faith-imagination prayer that specifically invites Jesus into the hurtful memories of trauma can invite a flood of healing grace.

How does faith imagination work? Suppose you feel stung and humiliated by what some colleagues said about you in a meeting. You might invite Jesus to return to the meeting room with you in your imagination. Opening your capacity for imagination as best you can, reexperience the awful meeting just as it happened but this time with an awareness of Jesus' presence. In your imagination pay attention to Jesus' reaction to the situation, trusting your perceptions for the time being and expressing whatever you feel. You might let yourself cry or speak aloud words of anger. Save evaluation of the experience for later.

Faith imagination does not require you to see pictures in your mind, although you might. You might *hear* Jesus speaking the truth to your colleagues, or he might tell you how he sees you. You might *see* him deciding to chair the meeting himself. You might *sense* Jesus wiping away your tears or leading you out of that room. Or you might be given a new way to *understand* your colleagues' behavior. Faith imagination does not attempt to reason what Jesus would probably do. Instead it invites the participant to an unpredictable encounter with the living God.

The perceptions that emerge during faith imagination create a *"healing icon"* of God's work in you, one you can return to again and again until you assimilate its message. These icons seem to be tailor-made for each individual and tend to offer exactly what each person needs at the time. Faith-imagination healing icons are particularly important when healing from trauma, for healing icons can begin to overshadow the horrific images and perceptions created by the terrible experience. (You will find examples of healing icons in the pictures scattered throughout this book.) Faith imagination can be compared with putting an old picture in a new frame; the entire feeling and look of the picture changes.

Persons who have not experienced faith imagination may object that it sounds like a process concocted from daydreams and wishes, all couched in the language of prayer.

They may wonder how you can know if you are perceiving a message from God or just entertaining a fantasy. That's a good question.

Faith-imagination prayer can certainly be distorted. All kinds of inner static—such as denial, old inner "tapes," and memories of parental injunctions—can prevent a person from perceiving clearly. That's why praying occasionally with someone else or with a group is a good idea. When inner static gets in the way, someone can tell you, "That doesn't seem like Jesus to me. Let's try again, shall we?"

Here is an important truth to remember: You cannot compel God with your prayers. Of course, sometimes when you pray, nothing at all seems to happen. At such times you learn to wait for God's timing and try again another day.

I am convinced, however, that God often uses faith imagination to get through to us. Evidence for this belief is the healing that occurs with so many people in often surprising and unpredictable ways. Faith imagination has long been a vital part of many healing ministries. You may recognize faith-imagination prayer in many stories in this book. For examples, see the stories "Healing of Terror" (page 117) and "Reminder" (page 128).

I urge you to try faith imagination for yourself as you work with the prayer suggestions in this book. See how God might want to light the way in your own life. Although we can seldom predict just how God will heal in a given situation, I believe that God wants to pour grace on you as you open your heart and mind to Love itself.

PREPARING FOR FAITH IMAGINATION

Before getting started, it is important to keep a few guidelines in mind:

1. *Remember that God wants to communicate with you.* God wants to heal you in some way (though not necessarily in the way you have in mind) and to lead you toward your own particular wholeness. God wants to show you personally how you can best love others and serve the world.

2. *Try not to be anxious about getting swept into feelings for which you are not ready.* Trust God to set the boundaries. Don't push yourself (or anyone else) to express deep feelings unless such expression comes naturally. If feelings pour out, possibly God is calling forth these feelings in order to heal them. A good cry or the honest expression of anger in the Lord's presence can be wonderfully healing. However, if you don't want to feel certain emotions, just come back to the present. It's okay to say no during the healing process. In fact, part of your healing may be to say a good, firm "No!"

To pull away from memories or feelings you don't want to experience, look around the room and name what you see. For example, "I see a red couch and a tan rug. . . ." Listen to sounds and name them: "I hear a phone ringing somewhere, and birds outside. . . ." Be aware of your body and what you feel physically: "I feel tension in my stomach, and my breath is going in and out. My legs are stiff, but my arms are relaxed against the chair." Splash cold water on your face, or rub your arm gently with a rough, wet washcloth. Paying attention to your five senses can help you return to the present.

3. *Remember that everyone imagines differently.* When some persons pray imaginatively, they may see images in their mind's eye. Others may hear sounds, and if images are present at all, they are wispy and indistinct. Still others may not see or hear anything, but they sense vivid experiences in their bodies. A few people may receive a sudden insight, a revelation that changes the contours of their inner landscape. Most of us use a combination of ways to imagine, and our imagination works differently on different occasions. Allow yourself to pray in your own imaginative language and in the way that God is being revealed to you.

4. *Remember that God has many faces.* For most of us, Jesus is the clearest face of God; stories of his actions on earth help us imagine him fairly easy. Inviting Jesus into our pain is a marvelous way to open to God's healing. However, for some people, even committed Christians, Jesus may be a problem when it comes to faith-imagination prayer. For example, women with sexual abuse histories may find his maleness scary. (Other abuse survivors may feel that Jesus is the only safe male.) Many other symbols of God's presence can be used in prayer: Christ, the Holy Spirit, God's light, Love, our Rock and our Fortress, Mary, angels, and so on. Even if the prayer suggestions in this book speak of Jesus as the focus of prayer, feel free to pray in whatever way seems right for you.

GETTING STARTED

The prayer suggestions accompanying each story often include invitations to pray with faith imagination. If you have never prayed this way before, I suggest you try it before responding to the stories. Some familiarity with the process of faith imagination before practicing it may enable you to trust more deeply that God sometimes heals this way.

Begin by setting aside an hour or so, and settle yourself with your journal in a comfortable space where you won't be interrupted. Invite God to shape your time of prayer and to help you have eyes and ears of faith. If you don't know what matter to bring to God for healing, ask the Holy Spirit to surface in your mind and heart whatever God wants to heal in you now. In silence pay attention to what occurs to you.

It is important to note that not all healing prayer concerns deep pain or trauma. Quite often the grace revealed in faith imagination concerns integration, empowerment, the release of control, or the surrender of dearly held prejudices. Healing prayer can take the form of confession or the discovery that God is calling you to something new. It can show you who you are, in contrast to what others may say about you. Remember, emotional and spiritual growth is a lifelong process, sometimes difficult but always wonderfully rich and nuanced.

When you decide what to pray for, express your feelings to God as honestly as you can. Don't "pretty up" the prayer with nice language or soften your real feelings. God knows what's inside you already, but you may not be fully aware of your feelings until you begin to express them.

Then invite Jesus (or some other symbol of God) to be with you in a way you can perceive. Invite him to sit with you in your prayer room, and allow yourself to imagine him there. Or, if you are working with a painful or traumatic memory, invite Jesus to take you back to where the incident happened. Ask him to accompany you to the childhood playground where you were excluded, to the bedroom where the abuse occurred, to the site of the accident, to ground zero.

Pay attention to what Jesus does and says. How does he bring God's healing? What does he say to you? What does he do? Let him direct the encounter, and try not to toss out anything as unimportant.

Notice your responses. Are you frightened, elated, leaden, resistant, joyful? Do you want to move closer to Jesus, or do you want to run away? Is your body tense and achy, or do you feel relaxed and at ease? As the encounter unfolds, keep telling Jesus honestly how you feel, and stay attentive to his response. Even though the two of you may not exchange words, let a "conversation" develop between you. Remember that Jesus may communicate through a gesture or look or through the quality of his presence. Your response may also be wordless.

JOURNALING

When you feel finished, record in your journal what happened. This step is important for two reasons. First, *you can better evaluate your experience if you have it in writing.* Certainly you will want to review it in a few days to see if it makes sense, if it sounds like the Jesus of the Gospels, and if it seems to agree with the wisdom of the church. You will surely want to ask yourself whether the prayer opened you to growth in grace and love or whether it just confused you. If you're not sure, consider consulting with someone wise and experienced in prayer, or simply let the encounter settle for a time. Remember, the possibility for misunderstanding is always present. At the same time, have faith that God really does communicate with human beings in order to heal us.

Second, *having a record of your own healing icons can be a wonderful help as you open yourself to a lifelong journey of healing.* It can be a tool for discernment and a comfort on bad days. It can remind you of where you've been and can illuminate your growth trajectory. As one who has kept a spiritual journal since my teenage years, I can enthusiastically attest to the value of journaling.

If you don't already have one, I encourage you to get a real journal in which to record your healing process. While an inexpensive spiral notebook works just fine, you can buy a lovely bound journal at a bookstore or gift shop for not much more. Having a private and special book is a good way to cherish God's gift of healing and to honor yourself as a child of God.

Using This Book

The following stories include a wide variety of faith responses to the events of September 11, 2001. Although the stories share the theme of God's faithful desire to heal, they reflect the roominess in Christian tradition for varying theologies and styles of worship and prayer, and they offer hope that we can learn from one another.

Resist the impulse to read the stories at a gulp. Instead read each one slowly, letting it speak to your heart. Before trying the accompanying prayer suggestions, remain open to the possibility that a particular story may take you in a different direction from what is suggested. Depend on the Holy Spirit to shape your prayer response as you wait in silence.

Make sure you take sufficient time with the processes suggested here. You will probably need at least an hour for most of the suggestions; some will take even longer. Perhaps you can set aside an hour or so once a week or make time for regular retreats or quiet days. Check nearby monasteries or retreat centers to see if you can arrange for solitude.

If you decide to try a prayer suggestion, do so gently, without pushing, and on your own schedule. Feel free to adapt any suggestions to better suit your desires and inclinations. You may want to skip around or to linger with one prayer process for a while. You may want to try a particular suggestion more than once. You may decide that some ways of praying simply are not for you.

Some suggestions invite you to explore deep feelings prayerfully. Go ahead if you feel ready, trusting that God wants to touch your pain and will keep closed the doors you are not yet ready to enter. Always stay aware of your right and responsibility to choose which suggestions you feel ready to follow and which ones are best left for another day.

If you are recovering from severe trauma, I strongly urge you to find a therapist and a spiritual companion if you don't have them already. If one person can fill both roles, so much the better. This book is not meant to substitute for therapy, but the prayer suggestions can be helpful in a therapeutic process, especially if your therapist does not share your faith. Praying about therapeutic issues can greatly speed your healing process.

Finally, this prayer work is especially rich if you practice it with a friend or small group. Reporting to this tiny "church" what you perceive with your eyes of faith can help keep you focused. Silence may also be easier if two or more of you work together. And, of course, you will have the advantage of mutual support in the context of praying for one another.

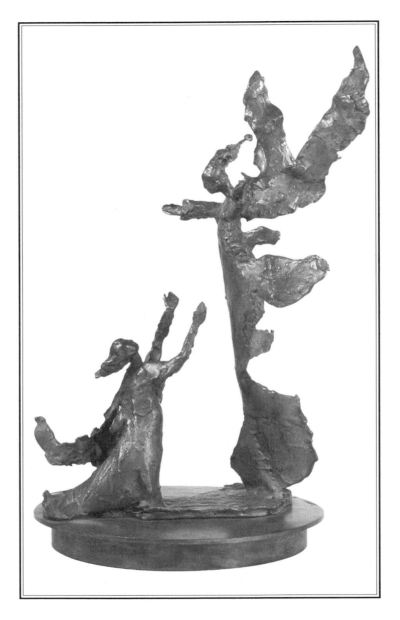

VISITATION

Tesia's Song

WANDA AND STEVE CRANER of Pottstown, Pennsylvania, were enjoying Disney World with their young daughter, Tesia, when the announcement came over the loudspeaker to clear the park immediately. No explanation was given for this unequivocal order. The crowd was simply told that it was extremely urgent to get to their various hotels right away. The mood of lighthearted celebration quickly turned to fear as worried parents hustled their children toward the exits.

Upon reaching their room, Steve and Wanda turned on the TV and watched in horror as news of the World Trade Center disaster flashed across the screen. Like the rest of us, they were transfixed and sickened by the unbelievable events. Coming directly from the fantasy of Disney World, they found the surreal images particularly disorienting.

As Steve and Wanda continued to watch coverage of the disaster, little Tesia wandered in front of the television screen, partially covering it with her small body. She began to sing softly, gently, simply.

Wanda was the first to let Tesia's song break into her consciousness. "Listen!" she said to Steve. "Do you hear what Tesia is singing?" With awe they listened as Tesia sang in her clear, small voice, her song expressing the prayer in their own hearts.

Tesia, not quite three, was singing:

Kum ba yah,* my Lord, kum ba yah.
Kum ba yah, my Lord, kum ba yah.
Kum ba yah, my Lord, kum ba yah.
Oh, Lord, kum ba yah.

Kum ba yah means "come by here." This song is an African-American spiritual.

PRAYER SUGGESTION

> Ask the Holy Spirit what song you need to sing right now. What song might God use for your healing? With what song might God invite your praise? What music might call you to deeper love and action? If nothing comes to mind, try looking through a hymnal or another songbook.

Sing your song, remaining aware of your need for healing. As Psalm 96 says, "Sing to the Lord." Let your song serve as a prayer that leads you into listening silence. When you feel you have finished, thank God for putting a song in your heart, and record your experience in your journal.

Admonition

MY SON, Noah Norberg-McClain, a graduate student at New York University, is a wonderful, gentle man whom I respect greatly. He does not, however, mince words when he has something important to say. As that terrible morning in September merged into afternoon, he saw me sitting shocked and immobilized on the couch, still watching television. He came into the living room and stood directly in front of me, blocking my view.

"What the hell are you doing?" he demanded.

"Watching TV," I muttered, hardly looking at him.

"Mom, why are you sitting here when there's a crisis going on? Why aren't you out talking to people and helping out in some way?" He had my attention now. Then he let fly with a question I still treasure: "Isn't that what you do?"

"Yeah."

"Then slap on that collar of yours and get out of here. Go find a way to do what you know you have to do."

Noah was absolutely right. I recognized that God had spoken to me through him. Although I seldom wear a clerical collar, I quickly put one on and went with my husband, George McClain, also a United Methodist minister, to the Staten Island ferry terminal.

At the baseball stadium next to the ferry, a medical triage unit was setting up to screen the less severely injured who would be brought from Manhattan. Other clergy from all over the island had converged there as well; and together with the doctors and nurses, we waited and prayed as we watched the huge billows of smoke rise across the water. Regular ferry service had stopped, but a few boats came in carrying exhausted police officers and firefighters who just wanted to get home. A smattering of refugees from apartments in Lower Manhattan arrived and left the terminal just as quickly. Although we spoke briefly to a few people, we didn't really have much to do. Slowly the realization that there might not be many survivors began to dawn on us.

Waiting at the ferry, I had plenty of time to reflect on Noah's blunt and grace-filled words. I heard in them a gracious invitation to do what I must and to be the person God calls me to be. In the days following, his words became a rudder as I steered my way as a minister and psychotherapist through a time of national crisis.

PRAYER SUGGESTION

❧ Ask the Holy Spirit to remind you of your truth tellers. Who encourages you to be your authentic self? When has God spoken to you through another person's loving admonition? Wait in silence for an awareness to surface.

In your imagination, listen again to what that person said to you. Is God issuing an invitation to action? calling you to repentance? encouraging you to risk growing a little?

In your journal, converse with God about it and ask for the grace to follow where God seems to be leading.

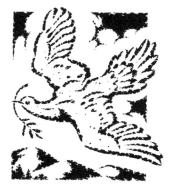

Assignment

Bob Lonergan, a former police officer, now works as a supervisor at the Civilian Complaint Review Board in New York City, an agency that investigates allegations of police misconduct. The CCRB office is located in Lower Manhattan a few blocks from the site of the World Trade towers. In addition to his work responsibilities, Bob is also a married Roman Catholic deacon.

Everyone in Bob's office heard the first plane hit, and some of the wreckage fell into the street directly in front of the CCRB. Immediately Bob evacuated his building and made sure everyone was safe. Minutes later when Bob saw the first building fall, both his training as a police officer and his identity as a deacon kicked in simultaneously. When everyone else frantically ran from the falling debris and choking cloud, Bob ran toward it. As a former cop, he could help direct the frantic mob; as a deacon, he could pray for some of the badly injured.

Bob grabbed a hysterical woman who was screaming and immobilized. As he took hold of her arm, she clutched him, causing them both to fall. Bob sustained a broken rib and a lump on his head, and the woman lay bruised and bleeding. Bob dragged her to her feet knowing that he could not abandon her; in her panic she would never be able to get herself out of the area.

In retrospect, Bob said that somehow he was linked to the woman at that moment. She was clearly "his assignment," as if God had sent him directly to her. Later he described his actions that day as prayer. Right then, however, was no time for theological reflection. He simply responded to an urgent need as a police officer and as a minister.

The two of them joined the crowd walking, running, and stumbling toward the Brooklyn Bridge, Bob physically supporting his much older companion and telling her she could make it. As they reached the bridge, fighter jets screamed over Manhattan, and the terrorized woman dived for the pavement. Later he discovered that she had survived World War II as a young girl in Bulgaria and still carried the memory of bombs falling around her.

While they were on the Brooklyn Bridge, Bob began to sense God at work. Even though badly frightened, people did not push and shove; instead, they encouraged one another. The black mud in all of their mouths made the crowd desperately thirsty, yet those who had water bottles shared them. Some Hasidic Jews handed out water, tissues, and oranges. As the crowd neared Brooklyn, Roman Catholic Bishop Thomas Daily stood on the bridge inviting everyone to rest in nearby Saint James Cathedral.

It felt wonderful to rest and cool off in the church. Bob and his companion, both filthy with soot, stayed for Mass before beginning a long, hot trek together on the Brooklyn-Queens Expressway, now eerily devoid of cars. Bob figures that they walked about seventeen miles that day. When his cell phone finally chirped into life, he called his sister and asked her to pick them up near the Kosciusko Bridge. It turned out that his companion, whose name he never learned, lived just two blocks from the school where his wife teaches.

As Bob reflects on that day, he is amazed at the many examples of loving action he witnessed. He also is moved by a resurgence of interest in matters of faith. As he speaks in churches around the city and helps lead ecumenical services, he sees a new spiritual hunger in people since September 11. "There is a lot of interest in discussion and faith sharing, especially among people in their twenties," he says. "God is using 9/11 to draw us back to a religious foundation."

Bob insists that he is not a hero. He feels that God sent him to help just one person, and the experience helped him as well. He calls his wife more often now to keep in touch. His faith has deepened, and he finds himself more drawn to silent prayer. Long walks on his lunch hour feed his spirit with solitude, even in the crowds of Lower Manhattan.

PRAYER SUGGESTION

❧ Bob saw God at work in the many acts of kindness from strangers and in his own actions. Ask Jesus to take you in your imagination to a time of fear and chaos, either from your personal life or to a scene from 9/11. Ask Jesus to show you how God was present in that situation. Ask what God was doing. Ask for eyes and ears of faith. Then wait in silence for an impression to form in your mind and heart. Respond, and ask more questions if you want. Have a conversation with Jesus.

Write about your experience in your journal.

❧ Go for a walk where there will be crowds of people, such as a busy street or a shopping mall. Invite God to alert you to someone who might need your help. What small kindness might you offer someone? Can you pay attention to the people around you while directing your heart toward God? Listen with your heart and, as best you can, respond to God's direction. Try to make sure you won't be recognized or thanked profusely.

How do you feel? What did you learn? Record your experience in your journal.

Subway Shrine

HIDDEN DEEP UNDERGROUND in the 14th Street subway station is an office of the New York Police Department. The Transit Police Bureau, District 4, is situated where large crowds of people stride by twenty-four hours a day with their heads down, intent on catching the next train or transferring to another line in the least possible time. Usually no one notices the police station; it is just another establishment down there among the newsstands, subway musicians, flower stalls, donut shops, and pizza-by-the-slice joints.

Since September 11, however, the police station attracts a little more attention. In front of the station and far down an adjacent side ramp, a large area has been cordoned off. An outpouring of cards, letters, posters, stuffed animals, fresh flowers, and candles has created a veritable shrine, a holy place of caring and remembrance.

Directly in front of the police station sits a large table covered with a blue cloth. Clearly a makeshift altar, the table is laden with remembrances and photos of two of the many people who died on September 11. On the table are teddy bears, Bibles, flowers, candles, a crucifix, and a picture of the Virgin of Guadalupe. "We love you Uncle Ray" is written on poster board in a child's handwriting. Someone copied Psalm

27:1-3 onto a piece of paper and placed it on the altar. Hundreds of cards and letters from all over America, many containing prayers and encouragement to trust in God, spill over the table and onto the floor, walls, and pillars.

Mrs. Maynard's third-grade class in Birmingham, Alabama, sent this simple message to New York City: "You are in our prayers."

Keri Blank from West Virginia wrote a poem:

To those who feel the pain and grief,
There is no automatic relief.
Keep the faith, we'll make it through,
And always know we'll pray for you.

Teenagers from Saint Catherine of Siena Catholic Youth Organization in Metairie, Louisiana, wrote individual messages on a large poster:

"From miles and miles away, united we stand, together we pray."

"People of New York, never lose hope. We are behind you all the way. I love you and am praying daily for you. Love, Kim Montelelone, age 15"

"We ♥ you and you are in our prayers. We understand the trouble you are going through and we admire you for your bravery! Just remember 'you can do anything with God who strengthens you!' I ♥ you all!"

One young person, whose punctuation and grammar could use some help but whose caring was unmistakable, wrote: "May God bless all those people that lost there life's and there kids."

A poster from Onsted, Michigan, proclaimed, "We love

you NY" above a hand-drawn cross. Underneath was lettered "Jesus wept" along with the citation of John 11:35, and a verse paraphrased from Jeremiah 29:11: "For I know the plans I have for you, not to harm you, plans to give you a hope and a future."

And finally, a long and anguished handwritten prayer signed "KD the Bronx, 9/15/01," excerpted here: "God of Love, God of Mercy, God of Peace, Our God, My God . . . Please God, don't take them all . . . For those who may be waiting still to be pulled from that awful pit, let your presence be palpable."

What is happening here? This subway shrine is one of many such shrines that appeared in New York City after 9/11, as if the impulse to create holy places could not be contained and spilled out of church, synagogue, and mosque onto the street. One shrine in front of the morgue on First Avenue grew so large that a tent was erected around it. There Protestant and Catholic services were offered regularly, and Jewish seminarians kept vigil twenty-four hours a day. Dario Oleaga, an artist who photographed many of these impromptu shrines, said, "New York became a single altar."[1]

Since September 11, it has become clear that the role of public prayer and proclamation does not belong solely to those with theological sophistication. Suddenly ordinary people have begun sharing their faith on sidewalks, walls, and lampposts, quite literally preaching to one another. Reaching out in love to passersby, people have created posters, poems, vignettes, and altars that call us to remember those who died and to remind us of the Holy One in our midst. Surely the Holy Spirit has once again broken out of the confines of established religion and shines through these humble messages found all over the city, messages born out of the faith that "God is our refuge and strength, a very present help in time of trouble" (Ps. 46:1).

PRAYER SUGGESTION

🦅 Create your own altar, asking the Holy Spirit for guidance. What will be the focus of your altar? Images of hope and faith related to the 9/11 disaster? Concrete reminders of God's presence and love? Symbols of your painful personal history or symbols of your healing? Reminders of things for which you are thankful? Pictures of people and situations to pray for? A symbol of something you are being called to give up?

In silence wait for a decision to emerge about where to put your altar. What space do you want to recognize as holy? Where do you usually like to pray?

Collect items to place on your altar. You may want to keep your altar simple, or you may want to include a profusion of symbols. Remember, this altar expresses your desire for God's presence, and you can change it whenever you want.

Invite Jesus to sit with you in front of your altar. Allow your imagination to discover how Jesus reacts to your altar and to you. Later, take a picture of your altar to keep in your journal. Record what happened for you during this experience.

1. Seth Kugel, "Documenting Humble Shrines of Private Grief," *The New York Times*, 21 October 2001, 6.

Brothers

Father Anthony Cowan, a Roman Catholic priest in Manhattan, heard about a remarkable act of love that occurred as panic-stricken people were running down the stairs in one of the World Trade towers. As an Islamic Arab from Palestine was running for his life in the surging crowd, he stumbled and fell. Paralyzed with fear and unable to get up, he was trampled within seconds by hundreds of feet rushing past him.

Then the man felt an arm on his shoulder and a voice speaking to him, "Get up, brother! We have to get out of here." Unable to stand because of his injuries, he felt himself being picked up. Again he heard the voice: "Brother, we have to get out of here!"

Half dragged, half carried down many stories, the man finally emerged from the building leaning heavily on his rescuer. As the injured Palestinian turned to thank the person who had carried him to safety, his eyes widened, for the person who had called him "brother," the man who had saved his life, was a Hasidic Jew.

PRAYER SUGGESTION

❧ Pray for the ability to see every person as your brother or sister. Then go for a walk or watch the news on television. Look into the face of each person you see and say to yourself, "She is my sister; he is my brother."

Is it a stretch to identify everyone as a member of your family? What about a homeless person? a surly teenager? a cantankerous grouch? an alcoholic who has passed out on the sidewalk? a driver with a bad case of road rage? someone from a different race, religion, or ethnic background? Does this experience move you to action of some kind? After writing in your journal, thank God for your brothers and sisters, and pray that you will learn to love more deeply.

God in a Tea Towel

ON THE DAY of the disaster, strangers beautifully sustained Michael Clarke, a businessman from England, and his wife, Sheelagh, a candidate for Episcopal priesthood. Michael was working in a building near the towers when the first plane slammed into the World Trade Center. Immediately he knew that it could not have been an accident, as it would have been too easy for a pilot to make the tiny maneuver necessary to miss such a tall, narrow building.

After the first tower collapsed, the billowing cloud of smoke and dust prevented Michael and his coworkers from leaving their building. Trinity Church, normally visible from Michael's office window, became obliterated by a black void that choked out all sunlight. He could not even see the opposite edge of the window ledge, just four inches beyond the window glass. Dust and noxious fumes began seeping through the air-conditioning system.

Trapped in the fearful gloom, Michael and his colleagues could only wait for the dust cloud to settle. Someone turned on a radio with live commentary on the disaster. As they listened to the horrifying news, thoughts turned to loved ones. One of Michael's colleagues, seven months pregnant, managed to call her mother in Brazil, who was watching the scene live on CNN. Despite repeated attempts, Michael could not get through to Sheelagh, at home in New Jersey.

Meanwhile, Sheelagh had seen the first plane crash on TV and frantically tried to reach her husband. Sick with worry, she prayed and waited. After what seemed like hours, the phone rang. Although Michael was unable to call New Jersey, he had reached his father in France, who now was calling Sheelagh to say that Michael was safe.

Relief! But a minute later the second tower fell. Because she knew that Michael was still close to the epicenter of the explosion she was watching on television, Sheelagh's worry returned. For more than an hour she heard nothing. When the phone finally rang, it was a work acquaintance of Michael's who just happened to be home that day. He told Sheelagh that Michael was using Instant Messenger to contact him. Even as he spoke to Sheelagh, the man reported that Michael was typing: "I'm safe. Please call my wife and tell her so."

Some two hours after the collapse of the second tower, the dust outside had settled enough that Michael and his colleagues felt they stood a chance of evacuating the area. Venturing outside, they made their way into the choking, acrid plume. All was eerily quiet. Michael did not run; as he points out, that would not have been the English way. Instead, he reports that he and his colleagues strolled calmly, through the two-inch thick blanket of dust, heading south away from the towers.

As he continued through the streets, he passed a small deli. The restaurant staff had gathered towels, aprons, and table linens and prepared a large vat of cool, wet cloths. These they freely handed out to anyone who needed them.

Gratefully accepting a lovely wet tea towel, Michael wrapped it around his face, and suddenly he felt himself enfolded in the care of those generous strangers.

Unlike many who were stranded in Manhattan that day, Michael managed to get home in record time. He took the subway to Penn Station where he discovered that New Jersey Transit was running continuous trains out of the city. In the words of the conductor, "Nobody needs a ticket today."

Michael returned home, dazed and covered with dust, clutching the tea towel. Although he and Sheelagh were deeply shaken by the experience, they have preserved the tea towel as an icon of God's faithful presence. It reminds them that even when every security dissolves in chaos, God is present as ordinary people find ways to care for one another.

PRAYER SUGGESTION

🦈 Michael's holy tea towel may remind you of the story of Jesus washing the feet of his disciples. Read the account in John 13:1-17, and imagine yourself in the setting. How would you respond to Jesus' invitation to let him wash your feet? How would you feel about washing someone else's feet?

If you want to try foot washing, ask a friend to participate with you in this experience. Prepare a basin, hot water, and towels, and perhaps some soothing lotion to rub on afterward. Together, slowly read the story in John as if it were written for you.

As you take turns washing each other's feet, stay aware of your feelings. Are you like Peter, uneasy about having your feet washed? What makes you uncomfortable? As you allow your friend to wash your feet, invite Jesus to wash anything inside you that is dirty, sore, tired, shameful, and calloused. Listen as your friend prays for you. How do you feel?

Switch roles, kneeling in front of your friend. How do you feel as you take Jesus' role? Pray aloud for your friend as you dry his or her feet. After a time of silence, discuss your experience and thank God together.

Write in your journal what Jesus communicated to you. Is there some part of you that Jesus might like to wash more? How will you continue to "wash feet"?

The First Casualty

FOR MANY YEARS Father Mychal Judge counseled and con-soled, celebrated and mourned, laughed and cried with the men and women who served as firefighters in Lower Manhattan. They came to love and trust him, for Father Mychal obviously loved them. He would go anywhere at any hour to respond to a need of one of his widespread flock. Many described him as a clear reflection of the Christ he served. Father Mychal, remarkable Roman Catholic priest, Franciscan friar, gay activist, and enthusiastic member of Alcoholics Anonymous, was also a beloved chaplain to the New York City Fire Department. On September 11 Father Judge, accompanying the fire companies as usual, soon found himself amidst the chaos and horror of ground zero.

It is not clear just how Father Mychal died, although according to some reports, he was leaning over to anoint an injured person on the sidewalk when some debris fell on his head. His body was discovered in the lobby of Tower One seconds after the collapse of Tower Two. The pressure created by the collapse of the adjacent tower caused an enor-mous vacuum and began the damage of the tower in which Mychal died.

Firefighters and police carried him outside where he was

pronounced dead by an emergency worker, the first identified casualty of the disaster. In shock and grief, they placed Mychal's lifeless body on a broken chair and bore him to nearby Saint Peter's Roman Catholic Church, where they laid their pastor and friend on the altar. A news photo of Mychal being carried in the chair has been called a modern *Pietà*.

Since all the priests of Saint Peter's had rushed to the disaster scene, no one was there to administer last rites. It is not clear what happened next. Some say those dazed, sooty firefighters and police officers anointed Mychal's body and administered last rites, using Mychal's own holy oil, found in his pocket. Others say they simply knelt and, putting their hands on Mychal's body, prayed for him.

Whatever the details, the firefighters and police took an unprecedented action for Roman Catholic laity: in their shock and sorrow they assumed the work ordinarily done by priests, that of liturgically shepherding a soul from this world to the next. Father Mychal, a faithful iconoclast, would have been proud of them.

Father Mychal had written a prayer that he prayed daily:

Lord, take me where you want me to go,
Let me meet who you want me to meet,
Tell me to say what you want me to say,
And keep me out of your way.

Mychal Judge gave his life for his friends. He did this for years before he died, and his death was in keeping with the way he had lived.

PRAYER SUGGESTION

☞ Memorize Mychal's prayer, and pray it aloud slowly. Stand up and repeat it until it gets inside you. As you say this prayer, allow your body to express it. Don't figure out how to do this; instead follow your body's lead. Let your arm make a gesture; let your head move in the way it wants; invite your legs and back and the rest of you to move in response to Mychal's prayer. In these movements discover a sacred dance that you can pray again. Dance your thanks. Write an account of your experience in your journal.

Prayers of the People

THE CHURCH of St. Paul and St. Andrew, a United Methodist congregation located on the Upper West Side of Manhattan, is chock-full of talent. Many of its members are professional actors, singers, dancers, stage writers, and musicians. Soon after the September 11 tragedy, some of these entertainment professionals produced in the church's small theater "a creative service of healing." The service, entitled "September 11: In Our Own Words," began with a particularly inspired sequence.

Imagine nine actors dressed in black on a bare stage, standing and looking directly ahead at the audience. To the left of the actors, three musicians—a pianist, violinist, and cellist—play softly. Six singers, also in black, stand silently on stage. The only light in the theater is a spotlight on the actors. One actor begins a first-person account of that terrible day, telling the now familiar story of the planes, the explosions, the fear of nuclear attack, the falling towers, and the deadly plume of smoke chasing terrified people down the canyons of Lower Manhattan.

As the narrator continues, another actor begins to pray, "Our Father, who art in heaven. . . ." Before the prayer is over, another voice begins, "Hail Mary, full of grace. . . ." Then other voices join in with the great Jewish prayer, the Shema: "*Baruch ata Adonai, Elohenu . . .*," as well as "O my God, I am heartily sorry . . .," and Muslim prayers in Arabic. Suddenly we hear prayers in many languages—Spanish, German, Yiddish, Russian, Japanese, Swahili, Korean—all at once, and finally the singers burst into a hymn, creating a great holy cacophony of prayer surging toward God. Surely members of the audience were adding their own silent prayers as well, for the actors had drawn us into a true "prayer of the people," and our prayers formed a powerful counterpoint to the tragic story still being narrated. The presentation marvelously demonstrated how naturally we humans call out to God when the world seems to fall apart, united by our need for the Holy One.

PRAYER SUGGESTION

🍂 Recall what you prayed when you first heard the news on September 11. Was it a prayer you memorized long ago? Was it a visceral prayer such as "Oh God, no!"? Pray it again, and this time feel yourself surrounded by the great chorus of prayer from all around the world. Remember how on the day of Pentecost, the Holy Spirit miraculously sorted out the languages of "Parthians, Medes, Elamites, and residents of Mesopotamia, Judea and Cappadocia, Pontus and Asia, Phrygia and Pamphylia, Egypt and the parts of Libya belonging to Cyrene, and visitors from Rome, . . . Cretans and Arabs" (Acts 2:9-11) so that everyone understood one another.

What happens to you as you listen with your heart to the differing styles, languages, and theologies of prayer in our world? Can you imagine these prayers as a part of your experience of September 11? As a part of this great choir, what do you want to pray now?

Write your prayer in your journal.

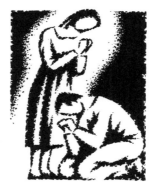

Painted Prayer

⌒

Virginia Laudano, a retired art teacher from New Jersey, now lives in Sun City, Florida. She lost a neighbor and six former students in the September 11 attacks. Three families she knows in Florida lost relatives as well. Overwhelmed with grief, Virginia experienced disturbed sleep riddled with frequent nightmares.

As Virginia met with her Roman Catholic charismatic prayer group one night soon after the attacks, a woman began to pray in tongues. As Virginia prayerfully listened to her friend, a beautiful picture formed in her consciousness, and she sensed the nearness of the Holy Spirit. She saw a sky of gorgeous blue parting to reveal a light-filled opening. Inside the opening, surrounded with radiance and tumultuous clouds, a dove descended. Angels flew toward a dark, undifferentiated landscape and rose toward the dove, carrying souls to heaven.

Virginia was astonished by the beauty of her vision and stunned when the woman praying in tongues reported seeing a similar image. Immediately Virginia knew she must try to paint what she had seen. The wonderful, peaceful blue of the sky particularly moved and challenged her. That indescribable color spurred her to capture what she had seen in prayer.

Usually when Virginia paints, she plans and sketches beforehand. This time she simply went into her garage studio and started painting on a large canvas. "It was pure inspiration," she says. "It just came, one, two, three. I felt that God was guiding my hand. It was unlike anything I've ever done before. It just bowled me over."

Virginia knew that the dark landscape in her vision represented the devastation of the World Trade towers, but the images were not clear to her. Only as she painted did the landscape take shape. In the shadow of the tower skeletons, she painted an angel cradling a single figure as light, emanating from the dove, rained down upon the ashes. But the painting was not quite complete.

One day Virginia saw a news photo of the Lower Manhattan site; workers had uncovered two huge girders fused together in the shape of a cross. Immediately she put this cross into the painting, finishing at last. "I didn't even want to sign it," she said, "because God really painted the picture with me." She speaks of that remarkable creative process as healing. "I was comforted and given hope," she says. "The whole thing reaffirmed for me that God was very present [in the 9/11 disasters]."

Not long after finishing the painting, Virginia was one of several people interviewed for an article on the resiliency of senior citizens. The article featured a photograph of her painting along with a brief explanation of how she came to create it. Right away Virginia began receiving calls from people all over the country who wanted to tell her how much her painting meant to them. A new ministry opened up for her as she listened with her heart to their stories.

Interestingly, many callers reported having visions similar to the one in Virginia's painting. Virginia mused, "It's a universal image, I guess."

To her astonishment, Virginia Laudano had created a symbol of hope. Like Russian icons of old, her painting draws the viewer in and invites him or her to discover a message. Her icon powerfully replaces images of devastation and terror with an image of God's love and faithfulness. The symbol so crucial in her own healing has helped many others.

How exactly like the kingdom of God.

PRAYER SUGGESTION

☞ Even though you may not be an artist like Virginia Laudano, find some art materials that appeal to you. You can use crayons, colored pencils, markers, or clay—whatever you feel most comfortable working with.

Invite the Holy Spirit to pray inside you as you experiment with your art materials. Don't set out to create a work of art; allow yourself just to play a little. Remain aimless and prayerful. If a shape or color emerges from your prayer, play with capturing it.

Did anything surprise you or catch your attention? Were you aware of God communicating with you? What happened for you?

Perhaps you would like to draw a picture to express your gratitude. Draw in your journal if you wish or describe your art play/prayer in words.

No Coincidence

THE SUNDAY AFTER the disaster I went to Snug Harbor, our neighborhood park in Staten Island, wearing a clerical collar and leading my dog, Phoebe. Wanting to be available to anyone who might need to talk, I figured that either the collar or the dog might break the ice. It was Phoebe that prompted a young man to approach me. "Beautiful dog," he said. "Thanks," I replied. "Do you like dogs?" And so we launched into a conversation that shone with God's presence.

The man said he was a carpenter, but since September 11 he had been out of a job. The person for whom he had been working lost a relative in the World Trade towers and had canceled her home-improvement project. Since then, the man had been aimlessly driving around Staten Island thinking about his life and what he wanted to do with the rest of it. A new inner clarity convinced him that his life had been shallow, selfish, and undisciplined. He felt different, he said, unsettled, and was entertaining thoughts he had never had before. He found himself visiting churches, slipping in at odd hours to sit in the silence without really knowing why. He explained that he used to be Catholic and until a few days before had believed that the church was simply irrelevant.

Now he was not so sure. He just knew that something was happening to him, although he couldn't say what.

And now here he was talking to me, saying things he had never told anybody. A little astonished with himself, he had no idea why he had stopped his car at the park and walked in. "I just did it without thinking. It's a real coincidence I bumped into you."

I replied that our meeting had God written all over it; in fact, it was as if God had arranged it. He smiled at that idea. Then his eyes bored into me and his voice dropped to a whisper. "What do you think is happening to me?" he asked. "Why am I feeling so weird?"

Usually I would not answer that kind of question directly, preferring instead to let people make discoveries for themselves. However, something about the intensity of the way he asked prompted me to answer him simply. "From what you're saying, I would guess that you're in some kind of transition to a new way of living and thinking about yourself," I replied. "All of a sudden you are looking at your life with new eyes. For the past few days you've been willing to be led by your intuition and hunches. I would call it the stirrings of God leading you to a different place. And it seems like a big part of this major shift is God drawing you back into a deeper and more mature faith."

I encouraged him to stay alert to what God was working inside of him and to take the ride. I further suggested that he talk to a priest about his experience. "But," he said, "is it really okay to come back into the church during a crisis? The priests are busy, and I don't want to go back just because I'm shook up right now." I assured him that it would be more than okay. He loved the idea of being in transition while God took him to a new place and of having a name for what was going on. He promised to stay alert and responsive to his inner process. Glancing at his watch, he said he had to go. "Thanks so much. This has been real good," he remarked.

I invited him to call if he wanted to talk some more; then he was gone. I think of him from time to time and pray that he will stay alive to God's nudges.

PRAYER SUGGESTION

🐦 Ask God to make you aware of divine nudges in your life. What has God said to you through recent incidents? What was God saying in that unexpected phone call? in that flat tire? in that moving television program? in that bout of anxiety? in that "coincidence"? In silence discover where God seems to be directing your attention.

Now pay attention to your hunches, your impulses. Obviously, not every hunch or impulse is a message from God, but God does sometimes choose to communicate this way. What do you feel an urge to do? Call an old friend? Take a nap? Go for a walk in the park? Read a certain book? Play with your kids? Offer forgiveness to someone who hurt you? Record your impulse in your journal.

If your impulse is not patently foolish, will not hurt anyone, and seems consistent with the gospel, try following it. See what happens. Discover what you feel. What other hunches are you aware of?

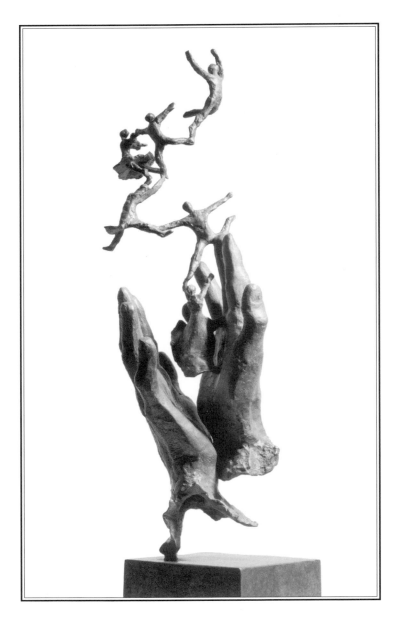

Healing in a Devastated Parish

HOLY CHILD Roman Catholic Church on Staten Island lost thirty people in the World Trade towers. Their pastor, Father Tom Devery, says that although September 11 is a day the world will remember, for him the hardest day was September 12. That morning parish members began to realize that their anxiously awaited loved ones might not be simply delayed by the crippled transportation system. Perhaps they were trapped under tons of rubble. And the worst thought of all: Their missing daughters, sons, husbands, or wives might never be coming home.

Family members of the victims streamed into the church early on September 12. Many were panicked, screaming, hysterical. Some hyperventilated into plastic bags. Others sobbed or were deathly mute. They came for help, for comfort, for a listening ear, for something to hang onto. They came for prayer when they themselves could not pray.

Ministering to so many people in crisis at the same time was an enormous pastoral challenge. Knowing he could not meet it alone, Father Tom quickly prayed, "What shall I say to them, Lord?" As he paused to listen for God's response, he recalled how Jesus had raised a twelve-year-old girl to life. Taking her hand, Jesus said to the dead girl, "Child, get up!" and the girl opened her eyes, restored to health (Luke 8:49-56). Somehow that familiar story from the Gospels shaped Father Tom's conviction that he must tell his frightened parishioners something utterly simple. He knew that his message would be "Jesus is with you."

"That's the heart of it," Father Tom told them. "Jesus is with you in your shock, in your anxiety, in your loss, in your grief, in your sadness and confusion. God is loving you through all of this. Wherever your loved one is, remember he or she is in God's loving arms. So trust in the Lord. Center in him."

The families had come to the church that day looking for hope. They wanted to be reminded of God's care, of what their faith could mean at a time of such profound loss. A few of them admitted they were angry and didn't want to hear any talk about the love of Jesus; all they wanted was for the person they loved to walk through the door. However, most of them gratefully told Father Tom later that he had given them exactly the message they needed to hear.

Out of the need to help so many anguished people in Holy Child parish, a new cooperative ministry sprang up between priest and laity. That same week the church began having Mass every night at nine o'clock, and despite the late hour, people came. Although the church's charismatic prayer group had never before engaged in such a ministry, they proposed to pray for individuals after Mass. Parish members eagerly availed themselves of this prayer opportunity, and God's healing mercy became evident to everyone.

With the faithful prayer group doing this important work, the priests were free to offer the sacrament of reconciliation (confession). Father Tom stayed at the church until after midnight most nights that week, listening as people confessed their sins. Many of the penitents had not confessed for years; some hadn't for decades. Father Tom sensed that most did not come to the church solely out of fear but out of a new clarity that saw the foolishness of holding onto guilt any longer. Old issues were being addressed; grudges were released; and attitudes were shifting. Even as the extent of the tragedy deepened in this congregation, members were already aware that God's healing love was moving among them.

The Sunday after the attack, six babies were baptized. Three of the children's fathers were firefighters who found it hard to muster a spirit of celebration for this important milestone. Though they were physically present at the baptism, emotionally they were still at ground zero, overcome with grief for their close friends and with guilt for having survived. As Father Tom gazed at the weeping men holding their babies, he said, "You have the whole world in your hands, you know." One father replied, "Yes, my daughter *is* my whole world." Then with visible new resolve he said, "I have to make the world better for her."

Another firefighter from the parish could easily have died but didn't. As he went up the stairs inside one of the towers, he noticed that his oxygen tank was empty. He turned around and walked out of the building to the fire truck, where he filled his oxygen tank. Just then the building collapsed, and the choking cloud descended. The fresh oxygen in his tank helped him breathe until he could crawl away to safety. Although he was grateful to God for sparing his life, he also felt guilty for surviving. In the immediate aftermath of the attack, he didn't see anything that could give his life much meaning. God, however, had a small surprise in store for him. One week later he and his wife, who had been trying to have a child for years, found out she was pregnant. Out of this man's devastation came hope and renewal, and most amazing of all, new life.

Another family in the parish lost both their daughter and son, one in each of the towers. At the memorial service there was loud wailing and "crying before the Lord." Family members did not hold back their devastation; they were perfectly comfortable bringing to God exactly how they felt. Watching them, Father Tom felt the nearness of the Holy Spirit, beginning the healing of this family's tragedy as they surrendered their tears to the Lord.

As Father Tom reflected both on the terrible tragedy and the powerful healing evident at Holy Child, he remembered his grandfather, a carpenter who helped build the *Titanic*. "It was supposed to be an unsinkable ship, and we all know what happened to it. We've been reminded recently that we can't depend on unsinkable ships any more. But we can depend on God, who is absolutely dependable."

PRAYER SUGGESTION

🕊 Ask a friend to join you for this prayer suggestion. Tell a story from your life, one or two sentences at a time. Your friend's job is to look into your eyes and tell you after each statement, "Jesus is with you in that." For example:

YOU: "My dad died when I was eight years old."
FRIEND: "Jesus is with you in that."

You: "He died of cancer. It was awful seeing him waste away."

FRIEND: "Jesus is with you in that."

Continue telling your story bit by bit in as much detail as you want. Pause after each statement to breathe in physically your friend's short "sermon." Another job for your friend is to remind you to breathe each time you hear that Jesus is with you!

If your friend wants to do so, switch roles. Give thanks together, and record in your journal what happened for you.

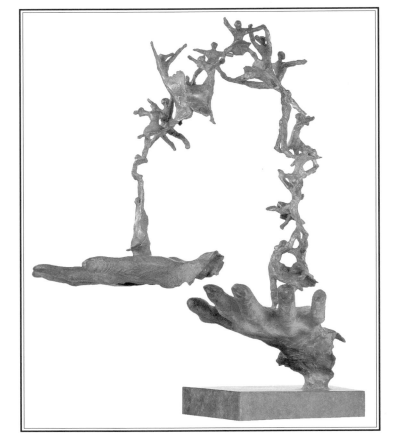

RAINBOW OF SOULS

Rainbow

Soon after the World Trade Center attack, Noel Koestline, a United Methodist pastor in Bayport, Long Island, joined other local clergy to plan an ecumenical service to commemorate the National Day of Prayer. They assumed that people would come to the service carrying shock, terror, anger, despair, and grief, and that they needed to recognize those feelings liturgically. The clergy decided that the service should suggest a movement from despair into hope. They wanted people to leave the service armed with hope, faith, and a sense of God's presence. The clergy did their best to plan for this movement and prayed that the service would be helpful to the congregation.

In the early evening just before the ecumenical service, a magnificent double rainbow hovered over Long Island. Among those who marveled at the beautiful rainbow were folks on their way to the service that Noel and her colleagues had planned.

After the service many persons shared that they had sensed God speaking to them through the rainbow. Seeing it, they felt better about everything; their fearful reactions to the disaster didn't seem so all-encompassing. Some articulated how the rainbow had reminded them that God's covenant promise remained intact and that they could count on God's love, no matter what. As with the story of Noah's flood, they saw the rainbow as a sign of hope and restoration.

The carefully planned service had burst out of the confines of time and space, beginning in a most unlikely place: the highways of Long Island at least half an hour before the announced time for worship. God had given the congregation exactly what the planners had prayed for: eyes of faith to perceive a grace-filled message of hope, comfort, and faithful presence.

PRAYER SUGGESTION

🐦 Spend some time getting in touch with what needs healing in you. How do you feel? What are you remembering? What feelings are you avoiding right now?

Now take this awareness outdoors. Ask the Holy Spirit to shape your attention so that you might see signs of God's grace, a "rainbow" for today. When an object or a person captures your attention, stop and allow the Holy Spirit to communicate with you. What does God say to you as you gaze at that beautiful tree? at that vacant lot? at the face of that child? As you encounter these "rainbows," thank God for each one. Record your experience in your journal, along with anything that has shifted for you during this prayer.

Anger Transferred

Dr. Larry E. Webb, a retired pastor and psychotherapist, left his home in Florida to come to New York as a volunteer soon after the disaster. Many people benefited from his compassionate listening during the weeks he spent near ground zero, and he was a godsend to the New York churches that eagerly used his skills.

One evening Larry attended a group at a church in which participants were invited to talk about their reactions to the disaster. He told the group that as he watched the towers fall on television, he experienced tremendous helplessness and a flood of tears. For several days he cried numerous times for the senseless loss of life, for the sorrow of the victims' families, for the trauma of a nation. He felt his tears were appropriate and good, and he let them flow freely.

During those same few days, however, another feeling began to run inside Larry. He was surprised to find himself angry, enraged, and vengeful. At first he thought he was angry at the terrorists, but he sensed that this explanation did not quite fit his feelings. He told the group that although he was not generally afraid of his anger, he did not usually react with anger to suffering, no matter how bad. Furthermore, he wasn't able to process this particular anger very well. It just stayed with him, always hovering in the background, ready to flare up at the least provocation.

Later in the group session the leader suggested faith imagination as a way to invite God into images and feelings generated by the disaster. Larry willingly invited God into his anger, but for many minutes nothing seemed to happen.

Then came a startling revelation. Breaking into Larry's consciousness like a sudden rain shower came the realization that this anger did not belong to him. Just as he had experienced in himself the helplessness of the victims and cried the tears of the families, he also experienced the anger of the attackers. Through the lens of his own emotions Larry caught a glimpse of how much anger the terrorists must have possessed to kill themselves and so many innocent strangers.

Larry was a little astonished, but somehow it felt true. As he made space in himself for this new understanding, he felt the anger that had been part of his life for six weeks begin to drain away.

PRAYER SUGGESTION

🐟 Invite God to give you the courage to stop discounting certain inner experiences. Ask for eyes of faith to identify God's work in thoughts and feelings that may seem a bit odd at first. Pray that you will cherish experiences that don't quite fit "into your box," as Larry did with his strange anger.

Ask the Holy Spirit if you have ever tossed out an important experience or hunch because you didn't understand it. Wait in silence for God to work in your heart.

If you receive an impression, write it in your journal

even if you think it doesn't make sense. Keep it in your heart, trusting that if it is important, God will teach you its meaning at the right time.

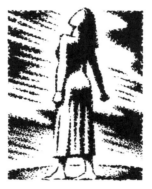

God Cleans House:
A Dream

FOR A TIME after the disaster, Elizabeth Braddon, pastor of
Park Slope United Methodist Church in Brooklyn, felt cen-
tered and calm, able to minister to her frightened congregation. She listened; she designed worship services; she
preached the gospel with faith and compassion. Folks from
her church had harrowing escapes on September 11; some
told astonishing stories about what kept them from going to
work that day. To everyone's relief, no one from her church
was lost. Like the fine pastor she is, Liz was there for her
parishioners as they processed these experiences.

All was not well, however. As Liz tells it, she had inter-
nally compartmentalized the fact that thousands of people
were dead. Although she did a good job of keeping the enormity of the disaster at bay, one night, several weeks after the
attack, it finally caught up with her. She was flooded with
so much horror that she could not close her eyes during the
entire night without seeing dismembered bodies and collapsing buildings.

A short time later Liz talked about that ghastly night
with Sara Goold, a colleague in ministry. Sara asked her if

she had invited God into the vivid images of mayhem that plagued her. Of course! That was what she needed to do, and Liz resolved to pray along those lines as soon as she could. Exhausted both from the intense demands of ministry and her personal struggle, Liz went to bed and had a dream.

In her dream it was night, and Liz found herself in the house where she grew up. The house was full of terrorists—not one Arab among them—who taunted, threatened, and scared her all night. When daylight finally came, the terrorists said they had to leave because they worked only at night. But they promised that they would return. They left, but Liz sensed that at least one of them was still hiding in the house, ready to kill her. Liz was badly frightened, and in her dream she asked God to come and cleanse the house. Although she couldn't see what God looked like, she felt certain that God was sweeping through the house, checking the corners and crannies, thoroughly chasing all the terrorists away. With that, Liz woke up.

Usually after a nightmare she feels tense and edgy; however, the morning after this dream Liz felt peaceful. Believing that God had worked powerfully while she slept, she felt a gentle, relaxed sense of "it's okay."

Not okay, of course, that the disaster occurred, but okay that God is surely stronger than the forces of evil. Okay that God can sweep away fear. Okay that God heard the prayer she was too exhausted to pray, and certainly okay that God chose to give her a healing icon in a dream.

PRAYER SUGGESTION

🦋 Before going to bed, invite God to be present with you in your dreams. Ideally, choose a time when you can sleep as long as you want the next morning; a retreat is a wonderful time for this kind of prayer work. Be sure to put paper and pencil beside your bed.

If you have trouble remembering your dreams, try waking up slowly. For a few minutes don't move; just allow your dreams to come with you into a waking state. As soon as you remember even part of a dream, sit up and write it down. Add as many details as you can recall, but don't worry if you can't remember the whole dream. Even a dream fragment can open marvelous doors to growth. Simply writing down your dreams may well help you remember more of them in the future.

To work with your dream, follow the prayer suggestion on page 89.

Aiden's Dream

NEW YORK CITY firefighter David Fontana's unit, an elite group specially trained in difficult rescues, was one of the first to be called in after the first plane hit. Immediately the company rushed over the bridge from Brooklyn. Every one of those heroes perished as the towers collapsed.

Big, sturdy, funny, loving David left behind his wife, Marian, and their little boy, Aiden, age five. At first Aiden couldn't believe that his daddy wasn't coming home again. He accused his mother of lying. While his mom prepared for a mid-October funeral, Aiden insisted on planning a big welcome-home party for his daddy. His denial was firmly and mercifully in place.

More was taking place inside this remarkable child, however, than denial. A few days before the funeral, Aiden had a wonderful dream that surely was a gift of God.

The antecedents of his dream are rooted in the previous summer when Aiden phoned his grandmother, Staten Island artist Joyce Malerba-Goldstein, asking her to draw a picture of an angel for him. Joyce quickly drew an angel picture and sent it to Aiden, who was thoroughly delighted with it. At first he insisted that his angel be hung over his bed, but it didn't stay there long. Aiden liked the sketch so much he took it down and slept with it. The picture's wrinkled tatters attest to how much Aiden still treasures the picture.

A few days after September 11, Joyce lay with Aiden on his bed as he prepared for sleep. "Nonna, I need you to draw me another angel," Aiden said. "It has to be big, with real big wings—big, big wings like in my dream."

"What dream?" Joyce asked. A psychotherapist, her ears perked up at the mention of a dream. What her grandson told her moved her beyond words. He said:

> The angel in my dream had big, big wings, and he is a very big guardian angel. He is watching me and Mom, and I saw Daddy with him. Daddy was with Jesus too, but he didn't have his fire hat on. Daddy was hugging Jesus a lot, and Jesus was hugging him back. I can't see Daddy now, but he can see me. I did fun things with Daddy. He played with me a lot, and he took me to the park.

Then Aiden told his nonna about all the activities he had enjoyed with his daddy. Before she left the room in tears, Joyce assured him that he would always have those good memories of Daddy inside him.

Joyce herself had a similar experience on the night David died, although no one knew then whether David was dead or just missing. While Joyce and I were praying together on the night of September 11, Joyce saw a clear image of David surrounded with golden light. This image comforted her enormously during the anguished days of waiting for survivors—or bodies—to be found.

PRAYER SUGGESTION

🐟 Before going to sleep, invite God to enter your dreams; put paper and pencil beside your bed. As soon as you wake up, write down your dream in the present tense. Include as much detail as you can remember. For example: "I'm in the house where I grew up. I'm cooking soup with Mom, peeling carrots, and there is a strange dog with us in the kitchen. . . ."

As soon as you have an hour or so, work on your dream. Here's how:

First, pray that God will shape your awareness. Then read your dream aloud. Understand that nearly every part of the dream represents a part of you: the house, the kitchen, the stove, the soup, the carrots being peeled, the strange dog, yourself, even Mom.

Unscrambling dream code is not hard. Don't try to analyze your dream; instead choose an image in your dream and playfully describe yourself as the person or object: "I am my old house. I'm not beautiful, but I'm warm and full of good memories. I need some repair; I'm full of clutter; and I have stuff in the attic that hasn't seen the light of day for years. . . ." Spend some time with this exercise. Do you find yourself saying something about yourself that rings surprisingly true? Do you discover anything about yourself? What might God be telling you? Try this exercise with all the objects and people in the dream.

Let images from your dream carry on conversations with one another. Let the dog talk to the house, or the stove talk to Mom. What can you discover? What changes for you?

Stay alive to the possibility that God might speak directly

in your dream images. Sometimes God is revealed clearly, as with Aiden's angel, but usually God images are disguised as ordinary dream images. Discovery of God's message in a dream usually occurs in the dreamwork of playfully becoming each object. In this simple process God's voice sometimes shines forth. For example, can you hear God's voice in the following bit of dreamwork?

"I'm a strange dog in your kitchen. You can shoo me away, you can forget about me, but I'll always be here. I'll never leave. All I want is to find my home with you. . . . "

If you don't "hear" God in your dream, invite Jesus (or some other symbol of God) to enter into your dream as you work on it. In other words, let your imagination make room for Jesus to interact with your dream images. What does he do or say in your dream?

Thank God for your dream, and record your dreamwork in your journal.

Grief, in Pieces

MARIAN AND DAVID FONTANA would have celebrated their eighth wedding anniversary on September 11, 2001. They had planned to spend the day together going to the Whitney Museum of American Art and lunching at the Central Park Café. Instead, David, a firefighter, got on the truck when the alarm sounded. A minute or two later he would have been on his way home. Marian never saw him again.

Understandably, Marian has been devastated with sadness. Sometimes just getting through the day has been unbearably difficult. Being both Mommy and Daddy to their five-year-old son, Aiden, while dealing with her own crushing grief has been terribly draining. Small frustrations that she could ignore before now stretch her tolerance to the limit.

Marian's faith in God has been shaken too. She had always felt profoundly grateful for the gift of David and Aiden. "I really didn't take my blessings for granted," she reflects. "I gave thanks to God for them every day." Marian says that her religion has been important to her in a way that was "very personal and quiet, expressed in living rather than in going to church."

Now after David's death, she can't help feeling punished,

as if she had done something wrong. She finds it hard to understand why God would take such a good man in the prime of life. God evidently saved some other people, so why not David? Naturally she is very angry as well. "Some people tell me it was his time to go, but I know in my heart it wasn't! And priests have told me it was God's plan for David to die. Well, that's a [expletive] plan! It sucks!" She is also mad at David "for leaving me with this big mess!"

Intellectually she knows that God was not responsible for David's death. She also knows that she is in too much pain right now to work out the theology of it all. Yet she wishes she could. "I'm almost jealous of my more religious friends. I wish I could have more faith. I'm having an intellectual battle with my spiritual and philosophical side." Wisely, she holds out the possibility that someday she will have more faith. "I know my old faith is working in me somehow and that I'll get it back."

Meanwhile, Marian finds comfort in the love and kindness of others, especially the other firefighter widows. And, in some measure, she draws on their faith. She speaks of one widow in particular, a hospice nurse, who has been with a lot of people as they died. "She is 100 percent convinced that when people die they go to a better place," Marian reports. "It's comforting to hear that, although most of the people who die in hospice are a lot older than David."

Like many widows, Marian talks to her husband every day. "I feel his presence with me a lot more than God's. Maybe for me right now it's the same thing. I just don't know."

Aiden is also a source of spiritual comfort. "Aiden has had a lot of angel dreams," she says. (See Aiden's Dream, page 87.)

"He has a lot of faith that has not been challenged by the death of his father. I'm glad he has it to hold onto. It's comforting to see him believing."

Soon after David died, Marian was propelled into an enormous new responsibility. Because she is feisty and not afraid to speak her mind, she quickly emerged as a leader among the families bereaved by the disaster. She now serves as the unpaid head of the 9/11 Widows and Victims Family Association. In that capacity she has been interviewed on television and is in direct contact with the mayor and other city officials. She was the subject of several feature articles in *The New York Times*. She has turned down Oprah twice. Her phone rings constantly with new requests and demands. She didn't seek out this role of running a large organization of wounded people with urgent needs; it simply snowballed around her. Sometimes the job overwhelms her.

This massive responsibility has forced Marian to rethink her professional life. Until 9/11 she was a comedian. Her one-woman shows, which she wrote herself, were quirky, smart, and funny. Now she wonders where to go from here. Although much busier than she would like, she is proud that her work has made a difference. Still, she is not sure where this new life is taking her. So much has changed so fast. Marian lives a day at a time, trying her best to meet the challenges as they come and to keep a stable home for Aiden. Sometimes she just doesn't feel up to the task. On days when sadness overwhelms her, Marian's good sense is evident; she cancels her appointments and allows herself time both to sleep and to feel the maelstrom of grief that is always with her.

At the end of our interview I told Marian, whom I have

known since she was a young teenager, that I had been praying for her. "Thanks," she responded. "I do believe in the
power of prayer."

PRAYER SUGGESTION

❧ In your journal make a list of your "pieces," parts of
your life that are full of stress, worry, uncertainty, fear, and
pain. If you are grieving, be sure to include that on your
list. For example, a list of "pieces" might read like this:

Mom's death—feel so sad

Why did God make her suffer so long?

Who will take care of Dad?

I'm so tired. All I want to do is sleep.

Should have told Mom I loved her when I had the chance.

Am I gonna be able to keep my job? What happens if I'm
laid off?

Where can I live when my lease runs out?

Always wanted to create art. How?

Can I go back to school? Money?

Write each item from your list on a small, irregularly
shaped piece of paper. Put your pieces on a plate (after all,
you have a lot on your plate!), and place it on your altar if
you created one. (See the Prayer Suggestion on page 53.)
Let it remain there as a sign of surrender and hope. Know
that you can't make your pieces fit, but God can bring grace
and healing in ways you can't imagine now. From time to
time, look at the pieces on your plate, and write in your
journal how God seems to be shaping your life in new ways.

Birthday

SAM IS A PASSIONATE twenty-year-old whose faith in Christ is the center of his life. A longtime member of Holy Child Roman Catholic Church on Staten Island, he finds special meaning in the parish youth group, Teen Catholics in Action.

Since 1999 Sam has felt called to some form of ministry; but on 9/11 he felt with clarity a more specific call to be a missionary. On that day Sam was mowing a lawn for a landscaping firm on Staten Island when he heard God say to him, "Sam, quit your job." "Quit my job! Why?" was his surprised response. Then Sam heard God speak the following words: "Do not worry. Be still and know that I am the Lord your God. I am with you. I'll never leave you or forsake you, for I have chosen you and empowered you with my spirit. Go and minister to my hurting people."

"That's when I felt a tugging on my heart to be a missionary. I quit my job on September 11, which happened to be my birthday, and got on my bike and rode to the ferry terminal," Sam says. Although untrained, that very day he set out to be a missionary, "to bring aid and God's love." Those who don't know Sam might call his action impulsive, even foolish. Some would say that first he should have engaged in careful discernment or gotten some training.

Sam simply says he was following God's call in the best way he knew.

Not everyone who wanted to help at the disaster site was allowed beyond the fence, but by September 12 Sam was working as a volunteer at ground zero. He says it was "the best job ever." He was there for six weeks clearing rubble, but quite soon he gained the confidence of his coworkers and served as an impromptu missionary. He came to see the site as "a great pain in a blanket of love," where "evil took over for a day, but where love prevailed. God was in every face I saw." Working at ground zero was a powerful experience that both began his training and further shaped his call. He is eager to finish his schooling so he can work full-time in the mission field.

Five months later Sam marvels at the gift he received on September 11, his birthday. He says, "God used me, a mere twenty-year-old kid who knows nothing about ministry, to help people."

PRAYER SUGGESTION

✔ Sam saw ground zero as a "great pain in a blanket of love." In your imagination go to a scene of great pain: a memory from your own life, a scene from the disaster of September 11, the Israeli-Palestinian conflict, or whatever. Trust that God will show you only what you are ready to see.

Let yourself experience the scene as best you can. What do you see? hear? sense? How does being there make you feel? What is happening in your body as you allow yourself to be in this place of pain?

Invite Jesus to join you there. How does he bring God's healing to the scene? Notice what he does and says. Do you sense a "blanket of love" around the pain? What happens to you as you remain there with Jesus?

Record your prayer in your journal.

☙ Describe your passions in your journal. How has God called you in your own life? What do you know you must do? Are you ready to say yes or reaffirm a previous yes? If so, let your readiness form your prayer. If you are not ready, be honest about it and let reluctance be your prayer.

Record your experience in your journal.

God Grieves

Dr. Robert Webber, emeritus professor of New Testament at Lancaster (Pennsylvania) Theological Seminary, is a man of deep faith, well appreciated by his former students for his excellent teaching and pastoral heart. Bob was watching television on September 11 when the second plane flew into the tower. He recoiled in horror, sickened by the awareness that this destruction resulted from human intention and ingenuity. "I call that intention evil, as all antilife power is evil," Bob says. "I felt almost an awe at that evil." That evil had an immediate personal impact on Bob, whose son lives in Manhattan not far from the World Trade Center. It was a long, agonizing day before he was able to make phone contact with his son and to discover that he was all right.

Bob says that for him the faith question that 9/11 poses is whether we will allow the actions of terrorists to turn us into terrorists. "And the answer my faith gives is no; we must not allow them to. Talk of wars, of good versus evil," he goes on to say, "is absolutely against the gospel Jesus taught and lived. The way we become 'children of our Father/Mother in heaven' is to love our enemies and pray for our persecutors. Why? Because that's the very heart of God, who loves and blesses equally those whom we label evil and good." These days Bob prays for peace and for people our nation considers enemies, believing that "we humans are made with two arms, and we can embrace people on either side of a division."

Bob deplores the rhetoric and behavior of war that "encourages terror and counterterror, the very cycle of violence happening in Israel/Palestine." He fears that the United States is doing what the Israeli government has done—"causing terror in the name of fighting terror, thus perpetuating the spiral of violence."

Bob is "in awe before the pain we humans continue to inflict on Love," and in this pain, Bob recognizes the suffering of God. "I think the perfection of God's love must mean that God's suffering over the brokenness of the world is also perfect—that is, limitless."

Now Bob's prayers consist of a willingness to be present to God's suffering. "God grieves, and for now my faith response is just to sit with God in wordless grief, waiting for a sign. I ask what God is doing today, and what God is calling me to do and be."

PRAYER SUGGESTION

🐦 Spend your prayer time just sitting with God. God can hear your heart's prayer, so let your words fall away. Still your mind as best you can, not by being stern with yourself, but by letting go. Relax your body. Let your breath come easily and deeply. If you get distracted, gently refocus by breathing a centering word such as *Jesus, God, holy,* or *peace.*

For now, you have nothing to do but be with the One

who loves you. Wait with peaceful attention for God to shape your awareness.

🐦 Do you feel drawn to grieve with God for the world? Tell God so. Sit with God quietly, waiting for the Holy Spirit to create any inner movement. Let God be in charge, knowing that you may have nothing to do but be there.

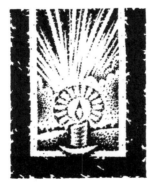

Icons of Choice

KAI CE BURTON, a psychotherapist from Collinville, Connecticut, was returning home from an errand when the planes hit. Shocked and horrified, she immediately called her husband, John, an Episcopal seminarian. Both were suddenly gripped with a vision that at the very moment of impact, Eucharist was being celebrated somewhere. On that awful Tuesday groups of people around the world had gathered in the name of Christ to receive once more the gift of Christ's presence and to be sent out to "love and serve the Lord." That morning brought Kai Ce and John the conviction that rampant hatred is always met by the power of Love—Love that transforms and cannot be overcome. Love that is stronger than death, stronger than fear, stronger than violence, stronger than hatred, stronger than cruelty. Love given to us in bread and wine shared around the Table.

The stark contrast between the terrible cruelty unleashed on September 11 and the radical Love that shows forth at the Lord's Table have become icons for Kai Ce and John of the choice we must make, both as individuals and as a nation. We must search our hearts for any characteristic that is not of God, for none of us is immune to the rage and vengeance that fueled the attack of September 11.

That is why Kai Ce passionately believes that the prayer that cries out to be prayed these days is one of contrition and confession. We must pray it for ourselves, she says; and we must pray it for our greedy, materialistic country. We must even pray it for the whole world, particularly on behalf of those who will not pray it for themselves.

PRAYER SUGGESTION

☞ Go to a Communion service, taking with you Kai Ce's realization that Communion symbolizes the vigorous, astonishing truth that nothing in this world can stamp out Love. As you participate in the service, remember that God's love is stronger than hatred, stronger than violence, stronger than disaster, stronger than political systems, stronger than death. Remember that Jesus initiated the Last Supper in the context of great fear and impending disaster, while evil was gathering force. Remember that Holy Communion is not simply a personal gift between you and Jesus but a sign that defies the "powers that be." When you pray the prayer of confession, pray it not only for yourself but also for the world. Thank God for what happens to you as you receive Communion through this wider lens. Write about it in your journal.

☞ Slowly pray the following traditional prayer of confession, making it your own. Pray it again, this time on behalf of those who might not know to pray it.

Merciful God,

we confess that we have not loved you with our whole
heart.

We have failed to be an obedient church.

We have not done your will,

we have broken your law,

we have rebelled against your love,

we have not loved our neighbors,

and we have not heard the cry of the needy.

Forgive us, we pray.

Free us for joyful obedience,

through Jesus Christ our Lord. Amen

Prayer taken from *The United Methodist Hymnal* (Nashville, Tenn.: The United Methodist Publishing House, 1989), 12. Used by permission.

Hospitality

WHAT YOU NOTICE first in Saint Paul's Chapel is the profusion of colorful cards, letters, banners, quilts, pictures, origami cranes, teddy bears, handmade wreaths, and posters that cover every wall surface of the large room, blanketing the back of each historic pew, climbing up the beautifully carved columns, and draping down from the graceful circular balcony. This amazing outpouring of love comes from all over the United States, indeed from all over the world. Saint Paul's has become a twenty-four-hour relief center for recovery workers at ground zero. The public is not allowed in, so the chapel is a genuine refuge for these tired, stressed men and women.

One poster brings greetings from the Cheyenne River Sioux tribe, proclaiming "*Mitakuye Oyasin*. We are all one family." Another poster from Münchberg, Deutschland, bears a hand-drawn rainbow over a dove carrying an olive branch. Underneath are the words, "*Vereint im Mitgefühl.* United in Sympathy." An enormous banner from Jesse Boyd Elementary School in Spartanburg, South Carolina, bears a cutout paper hand from each child in the school. Approximately five hundred pink and red hands are arranged in the shape of two concentric hearts.

A musician softly plays a good blues guitar, and the smell of delicious food and coffee wafts about the old building. Police officers and firefighters sit in the pews, chatting, eating, sleeping, praying. The chapel exudes an air of peace, order, and welcome. Volunteers quietly go about their business. A priest in jeans and clerical collar sets up for noon Eucharist. Fresh flowers and glowing tea lights decorate long tables covered with free items for the workers. In addition to the natural light streaming in through the soaring windows, the chapel is lit by twelve magnificent crystal chandeliers.

Saint Paul's has a remarkable history. It was built in 1766 as a chapel of the even older Trinity Church about a half-mile to the south. George Washington worshiped at Saint Paul's and attended a service of thanksgiving there the day he was inaugurated president of the United States. Soon after Saint Paul's was built, a disastrous fire destroyed much of what is now Lower Manhattan, including the original building of Trinity Church. Saint Paul's escaped damage and served as a refuge center for workers while the mess was cleaned up. No one could have guessed that three hundred years later, Saint Paul's would offer hospitality again under astonishingly similar circumstances. Although Saint Paul's is located directly adjacent to ground zero, the chapel sustained little damage on September 11 and emerged as one of the few intact buildings in the restricted area.

In recent years, Trinity Church had been pondering what to with Saint Paul's Chapel, which has no congregation of its own. A few services, concerts, and civic events were held there, and of course people came to see George Washington's pew, but that hardly seemed an adequate use of such a glorious space. Trinity Church was actively searching for a ministry for Saint Paul's when this astonishing ministry landed on its doorstep. Trinity Church has been running to catch up with God's leading ever since.

The new ministry began with a daily "barbecue on Broadway," a sidewalk operation to feed the hundreds of police and firefighters at ground zero. Soon it grew into a full-fledged feeding center for rescue workers. Seminarians, staff from the The Seamen's Church Institute, and volunteers from other parishes in the city kept the project going during the early weeks right after the disaster. Within days the meal project moved into the church sanctuary and was taken over by volunteer restaurateurs. The rear of the sanctuary became an impromptu cafeteria, providing free meals for rescue workers around the clock. For a while chefs from the Waldorf-Astoria Hotel did the cooking, serving as many as three thousand meals a day. Five months later, local restaurants supplied food to the church at a reduced rate, still dishing up about twelve hundred meals every day.

Early on it became apparent that the men and women needed more than just food. With no time for extensive committee meetings or to follow established procedures, Trinity Church tried to respond to needs as they surfaced. In the process this new ministry at Saint Paul's simply mushroomed. When some volunteers noticed that many workers were falling asleep in exhaustion, stretched out on the pews, they brought in cots and blankets and placed them in the sanctuary and balcony. And when they saw workers with cut feet and sprained ankles, church members made available boots, socks, and first-aid supplies. George Washington's enclosed pew space became a makeshift podiatry office, constantly staffed by volunteer podiatrists. A massage area, open twenty-four hours a day, was set up next to the ornate pulpit and cordoned off by portable room dividers. Clergy and other counselors were always available for counseling, and Eucharist was offered daily. Piles of books on grief and devotional materials related to the disaster were set out for the taking. Donations of candy bars, cough drops, soap, toothbrushes, face masks, work gloves, lip balm, warm hats, and a multitude of other items poured in and were placed on tables around the room. Ice machines, coffeepots, and free soda machines also found their spots in the church. Churches and individuals from near and far sent in donations to cover the costs. Letters from children around the country delighted the workers, who picked them up to read and sometimes to answer.

Outside the church, large canvas drop cloths were hung daily on the iron fence. Volunteers handed markers to passersby who might want to write something, and write they did. Clearly meeting a need, several drop cloths were filled every day with prayers and thoughts from the public. Along the way, a system of volunteers from churches around the country was organized; parishes clamored to get on the schedule to serve twelve-hour shifts for a few days at a time.

Recognizing God's hand in all this was not difficult. Not only did the chapel meet some of the physical, emotional, and spiritual needs of recovery workers, it also changed the lives of volunteers. They caught a vision of church that may greatly differ from anything they had ever encountered. They experienced a ministry of servanthood firsthand. They took back to their own parishes the memory of a church that valued people more than a building, even an old building of great historical significance.

Many parishes make a museum out of their church, protecting carpets and kitchens from outside groups. In contrast, Saint Paul's Chapel is a museum that has again become a genuine church.

PRAYER SUGGESTION

❧ How did you feel as you read about Saint Paul's Chapel? Were you moved and excited? a little shocked? Did you feel they should have found somewhere other than a church sanctuary to set up the food service? How do you feel about massage in church? Write your reactions in your journal.

Now playfully imagine what might happen if your own church decided to practice hospitality in a similar way. How would it look? What kind of hospitality does your community most need? Whom would you serve, and what resources would you need? Who might be interested in helping? What hindrances would you expect to encounter?

Ask Jesus to enter into your playful imagining, and discover how he reacts to it. What does he communicate to you? Remember to record your experience in your journal.

The Whole Picture

BETTE JOHNSON SOHM of Staten Island was looking at a list of the names of disaster victims when she discovered that she knew two of the passengers who died in the plane crash in Pennsylvania. One was a well-liked former boss, and the other had been a work colleague years before.

Suddenly catapulted into a personal relationship with the tragedy, Bette recoiled in shock. Almost immediately she began to imagine their last hours on the plane. Terror, helplessness, disbelief, paralysis, and horror filled Bette's consciousness. In her vivid imagination she could hear the noise of the engines and the chaos of screams and wailing mingled with prayers. She could feel the panic in her own body. She could see weeping people huddled together, holding each other. Emotionally, Bette was on the plane with them, and there she stayed for days.

I knew there was no use in trying to distract her from her inner images. A natural response to disaster and, indeed, part of the healing process is the desire to find out what happened. We need to know the details, even if the knowing is terrible. When the real story cannot be fully known, then invariably we create our own images, emotions, and sounds that give sequence and shape to the event.

Bette bravely faced what her mind and heart were telling her, but she could not move beyond it. A United Methodist lay speaker, Bette believed the promises of her faith, but she couldn't lay hold of them right then.

I suggested a faith-imagination prayer in which she might invite Jesus to join her on the plane with her two friends. As she prayed, it seemed that Jesus showed Bette an image of her two friends holding and comforting each other. They were praying, and although fearful, they seemed to have no sense of certain death.

Suddenly Bette saw nothing, as if her movie of the plane simply turned off for a few seconds. Then as her images resumed, she saw the plane in pieces on the ground. But in contrast to the cacophony inside the doomed plane, there was great silence and a surprising peace. Now Bette saw Jesus at the crash site in two different scenarios. In one image, Jesus was weeping over those who had died. In another, Jesus was saying to the people, "It's over, and you got through it. Your fear is gone. Your terror is a thing of the past. You will not have to suffer any more." And she saw him gathering up the passengers to take them home.

The effect on Bette was immediate. Although her image of the plane's last hours lingered, now she saw it through the lens of Jesus weeping and taking the people home. It was as if she saw the whole picture for the first time, and the whole picture offered deep comfort. She was no longer immersed in unmitigated horror but in the Light that shines in the darkness and is not overcome.

PRAYER SUGGESTION

🐟 Perhaps you carry a disturbing picture in your heart but are trying hard not to see it, just as Bette did. It might be an image from 9/11, or it might be the result of a personal incident. Ask God to help you to take a good look. Remember that you will not experience anything that is not already inside you. Remember also that Jesus will accompany you wherever you may need to go.

As you pay attention to your "inner movie," allow yourself to feel whatever emotion surfaces. Remember that crying or making other noise often accompanies the healing process. Then ask God to show you the whole picture, evidence of God's healing, grace-filled presence. Open your imagination so that you can perceive Jesus in your scenario. What is Jesus doing and/or saying? What message does his presence convey? Wait in silence and expectation for what God might reveal to you. Thank God for continuing to heal you, and describe your experience in your journal.

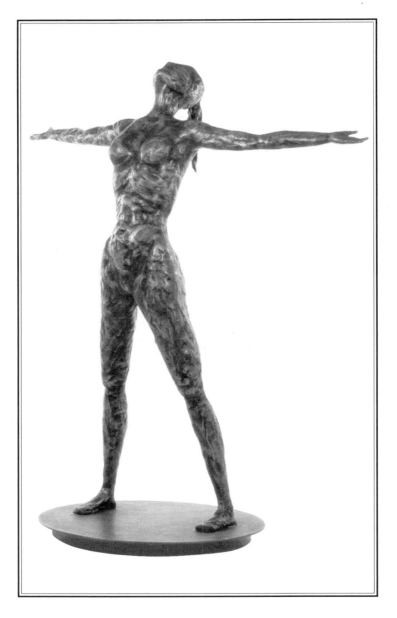

EMBRACE OF LIFE II

A Ritual of Healing

THE SATURDAY AFTER the 9/11 disaster, I was slated to lead a workshop on healing rituals at Fishkill United Methodist Church in Fishkill, New York. The date had been set for over a year, and I was prepared well in advance with a lecture and plan for an experiential workshop.

Obviously after the attack I had to revise everything. No one would be able to think of anything except the horrible event. Participants—myself included—would feel ragged and raw, and they would attend the workshop with hopes of drawing water from the well of faith. What could I do to help open all of us to God's healing? As I prayed ahead of time, I remembered some visits to the Taizé monastic community in France. Immediately I knew I would adapt the Taizé ritual of prayer around the cross.

The day of the workshop, eighty people showed up instead of the forty who had registered, revealing deep hunger for God in a time of shock and grief. I told them how the same healing grace that is poured out in the laying on of hands is also present in corporate rituals designed around a specific need. I talked about how Christian ritual "preaches" to the hearts of people of faith. I said that I believed that God was already working to redeem the awful tragedy and explained that we would participate in a liturgy that might help us open up to God's healing process.

In preparation for our healing ritual, we spent some time sharing our reactions to September 11; most were eager to tell how the tragedy had impacted each of them. Then I invited participants to answer the following questions in a sentence or two:

What image from television or newspaper do you carry? Out of the horror, what story particularly haunts you? What scenes have you imagined about the disaster?

In response, some spoke of bodies falling from the sky. Others mentioned the crashing planes and the proud towers collapsing like toy blocks. Many could not stop imagining the last few hours of the people on the doomed flights.

With these images tearing at us, we entered the church sanctuary for the healing liturgy. Communion elements were ready on the altar. A large pottery bowl filled with rolled washcloths for foot washing sat nearby, along with pitchers of steaming water. A life-sized cross lay on the floor.

The service generally followed the familiar liturgy for Holy Communion with some important additions aimed at our need for healing, beginning with the proclamation of God's Word. The New Testament reading was Paul's ringing declaration of faith in God's victory found in the eighth chapter of Romans, ending with:

> For I am convinced that neither death, nor life, nor angels, nor rulers, nor things present, nor things to come, nor powers, nor height, nor depth, nor anything else in all creation, will be able to separate us from the love of God in Christ Jesus our Lord. (8:38-39)

Instead of preaching a sermon, I invited participants to stand and find a partner; one would speak and the other would listen. I encouraged the partners to look into each other's eyes as the speaker paraphrased Romans 8:38-39. "Listen!" a speaker would say. "I am convinced that neither crashing planes, nor falling buildings, nor terror, nor terrorists, nor fires, nor rampant evil, nor anything else in all creation will be able to separate us from the love of God in Christ Jesus our Lord." The speaker would wait in silence for the listener to breathe three times, giving the listener time to take in the words. Then the partners switched roles, with the new speaker naming other components of the 9/11 disaster, ending with ". . . nor anything else in all creation will be able to separate us from the love of God in Christ Jesus our Lord." There was time enough for each person to experience this small "sermon" with eight or nine partners.

"You now have the opportunity to lay your burden on the cross," I told them. "That's where these terrible images belong. That's where your fear and sorrow can be held. Prayer around the cross says that you can't handle this alone. You are not big enough to carry so much horror in your soul. You are not big enough to contain so much evil, but here you can pray that evil will be contained. As a sign of surrendering your burdens, come to the cross on the floor when you are ready, and touch it in some way. Stay as long as you like."

In the long silence that followed, most of the participants found a place around the cross. Some touched it briefly with their fingertips before returning to the pew; others prostrated themselves in front of it for several minutes. God's presence was palpable as many wept tears of relief.

After Communion we washed one another's feet as yet another sign of Jesus' desire to wash and heal us and of our calling to be agents of this healing for one another.

In the next few weeks I used this ritual with several other groups. Each time participants reported being less anxious, more peaceful, better able to pray. A few reported they stopped having 9/11 nightmares immediately afterward. Now, alongside the horrific images, they had new images of healing and hope. God had worked powerfully in the liturgical actions that engaged body, emotions, and spirit to begin the process of healing.

PRAYER SUGGESTION

🕊 Adapt any part of this ritual for use with a friend. Paraphrase Romans 8:38-39 for each other. Wash each other's feet. Make a cross from sticks or scrap lumber; then surrender your burdens to Jesus through a gesture of touching the cross as you pray. Pause often so that you can assimilate what God is giving you, and thank God for the gift. Afterward describe your reactions to the ritual in your journal. What did God communicate to you through it?

Healing of Terror

SARA GOOLD, a United Methodist minister and psychotherapist, was walking in Lower Manhattan on her way to visit a friend on the morning of September 11. The spectacle of the burning, falling buildings was horrifying enough, but when she began to hear car radios broadcasting the news that the Pentagon also had been hit, she felt certain that a nuclear war had begun. Feeling utterly alone and terribly frightened, Sara wanted more than anything to be with her family. Her husband, Reverend Ed Horne, was in midtown that day at a meeting, and their young children, Olivia and William, were in school on Long Island near their home. To Sara, they might as well have been on the moon. Not knowing if she would survive to see her family again, she began to walk uptown numbly and automatically, in a sea of terrified people.

She found Ed at Christ United Methodist Church on Park Avenue with the church's pastor, praying and watching the surreal events on television. It was a wonderful relief to be with Ed, but neither Sara nor Ed could rest until they were reunited with their children. They managed to get a train home later that evening and finally arrived home safe but badly frightened.

Ordinarily Sara has a vital and sustaining prayer life, but in the following days she found herself almost unable to pray. The terror she had experienced just seemed to stick to her soul. It kept her awake at night and intruded into her work. A new fear of bridges and tunnels and a generalized low-grade terror kept her from attending a meeting with close friends a few days later. Even though she had looked forward to this meeting, she could not bear the thought of being separated from her children again.

Instead of going to the meeting, Sara stayed home and prayed. Or, more accurately, she allowed a prayer to unfold within her. Almost immediately she felt a deep sense of inspiration, a certainty that God was directing her mind and heart. She saw an image of Jesus gazing at her; he had dark, curly hair and a beard. As Sara looked at Jesus, she found herself speaking aloud words that seemed given to her by the Holy Spirit: "When Jesus called his disciples to follow him, they came because he loved them. Their response was not forced; it was not preordained; it wasn't a 'good sell.' They were drawn by his love alone. He loved them while he taught, and he loved them through the crucifixion. He loves us. He still loves us."

In the silence that followed, those words of love crowded out Sara's terror. At that moment she knew that Christ's love was more important and more real than anything else in the world. The prayer restored in her what she called "a sense of ground." It helped her recall that terrorists have been around for centuries, and that through the ages, during times of great fear, people have been able to stay rooted in the love of Christ. She would continue praying for grace to do the same.

Her prayer finished, Sara sipped a cup of tea. Suddenly she felt extremely tired and a little feverish.

Sensing that her body was finally letting go of the terror she had been carrying, Sara went to bed and slept it off. When she awoke hours later, her fear was largely gone, replaced with a profound sense of the love of Christ.

PRAYER SUGGESTION

🖙 Ask Jesus to open the door to something that frightens you. Perhaps you are anxious about your health or afraid that something bad will happen to a loved one. Maybe you fear public speaking or being in crowds of people. Maybe you harbor a memory that scares you, or perhaps you avoid certain emotions.

In your imagination enter the situation that causes your fear, and invite Jesus to be there with you. Allow yourself to feel your fear. What happens to your body? Does your stomach knot up? Do you tense certain muscles? Do you curl up or get ramrod straight? Do your hands sweat? Does your throat close? Does your heart beat faster?

Give a voice to some part of your body that is expressing fear. See yourself as that body part. You can either speak aloud or write in your journal. For example, "I am Sally's stomach, and I'm all knotted up. I'm crunching into a little ball, and I'm hurting—a lot. I'm trying to keep Sally small so she won't be hurt again . . ."

Now pay attention to Jesus. Watch, listen, and feel what he does. Discover how he brings grace to your fear. What is happening to your body now?

Remain in silence with Jesus until you feel finished. Thank him before you record your experience.

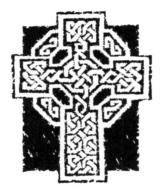

Nothing Can Separate Us from the Love of Christ

CAPTAIN SCOTT LAPIEDRA of the New York Fire Department, a married man with four children, died a slow, painful death as a result of his burns in a fire that occurred on June 5, 1998. His funeral was held in Saint Paul's Roman Catholic Church on Staten Island. In the midst of her terrible grief, Scott's wife, Addie LaPiedra, had a distinct impression of Scott being welcomed to his new life by Jesus. In her mind's eye she saw her exhausted and sooty husband, dressed in his fireproof suit and hat, being tenderly embraced by Jesus. This image was deeply comforting and gave her something to cling to as she grieved for Scott.

Addie decided that this blessing needed to be shared. In consultation with her friends at Saint Paul's, she and the church commissioned Canadian artist Neil Cox to create a life-sized sculpture of Scott and Jesus to be placed in the churchyard. To pay for it, the church would sell one thousand smaller copies of the sculpture.

It was a big project and a big risk. Would the church be able to sell enough of the smaller statues to recoup their costs? Nevertheless, in faith the model was sent to the foundry in the spring of 2001. At that time no one could have anticipated how excruciatingly relevant the statues would be when the casting was complete.

Summer had merged into a warm, beautiful September when the first fifty sculptures were delivered. Then on September 11 the unthinkable occurred, and Saint Paul's opened a twenty-four-hour relief center for rescue workers and grieving families. One of the new statues was placed on a table just outside the chapel.

Suddenly the little statues were in great demand. Whenever there was a firefighter funeral on Staten Island—and there were many after September 11—the family was presented with a statue. Other statues were snapped up by friends and relatives. Decimated fire companies, stunned with loss, wanted statues for their firehouses.

The statues are eloquent sermons about hope and faith in eternal life. Some people see their own faith images embodied in them. Others simply find them a great comfort. The little statues speak to grieving hearts of God's tender love, which extends beyond death. The fact that God used the tragedy of Scott LaPiedra's death to bring comfort and healing to countless others has not escaped notice.

The life-sized statue of Jesus embracing Scott was installed on the church lawn and dedicated on December 1, 2001, in memory of the 78 Staten Island firefighters who died on 9/11. (There are also plans to install a plaque in memory of the other Staten Islanders—nearly 200 of them—who died in the attack.) The words *No greater love* are inscribed on the base. Flowers and two benches surround the statue.

The statue of Scott and Jesus has become a pilgrimage destination for mourners and a light in the darkness of tragedy. It stands as a powerful testimony to the faith that nothing, not even the worst we can imagine, can separate us from the love of Christ.

PRAYER SUGGESTION

☞ What tragedy or suffering impacting your life might God want to use to help others? Can you even imagine finding blessing in your sorrow at this point in your healing process? Don't worry if you can't; trust that God can. Without making a blueprint, ask God to turn your suffering into gift. Thank God ahead of time for God's work. Record your prayer in your journal.

The Accident

⌒⌒

SOON AFTER 9/11 two drivers, one white and the other black, were involved in a minor traffic accident. The details of the accident itself aren't important to this story; all you need to know is that one car rammed into the other and made a big mess in the roadway, with crumpled fenders, bent doors, and broken glass everywhere.

Neither driver was seriously hurt; but with nerves frayed since 9/11, this accident stressed both persons to the breaking point. The man whose car was hit emerged from his car fighting mad and yelling; the other man grew angrier by the minute. As tension and volume increased between the two, uneasy bystanders gathered. Although their anger was unrelated to race, all the makings of an ugly racial incident were present.

Then abruptly, it was as if someone had pushed "pause." Both men stopped shouting at the same moment and just stared at each other in unmoving silence. Then light dawned: *They were alive! No one was hurt! Cars are just things! The other man is a human being just like me!*

Spontaneously they fell into each other's arms sobbing. Black arms intertwined with white ones as each greeted and comforted his brother.

PRAYER SUGGESTION

❧ Look through a current newspaper. Read three or four articles that capture your interest, staying aware of your feelings. Be as honest as can. Do you want to anesthetize yourself to the pain of the world? Do you avoid articles about conflict? Do you get a bit angry? Do you want to teach someone a lesson? Do you feel superior to or judge someone? Do you want to rescue everybody single-handedly? Own up to your reactions enough to write them down. Try exaggerating them on purpose in your journal so you can experience them more fully. For example, "I will *never* read those war stories. They're all the same—awful. I'll stick to the comics. . . ."

Then ask Jesus to help you see each story through his eyes. Invite him to show you how to push "pause" so you can see what is really important. Ask him to transform any of your attitudes that are not Christlike. Record any awareness that may come as you sit in silence and thanksgiving.

Intercessor

SUSAN RETHINASAMY, age six, is already a veteran intercessor. Every morning and evening since she was four years old she has prayed for others. Born in India, she now lives with her parents in Queens, New York, where her father pastors a Tamil-speaking congregation.

After September 11 Susan's faithful prayers intensified. No one had to tell her to pray in response to the devastation; prayer just came naturally. Every morning as her father drives her to school, she prays for those who survived the attack, as well as for the ones who perished. She also prays for the families of the victims, especially for the many children who lost parents. At this writing, five months after the attack, little Susan is still holding the September 11 disaster in daily prayer.

PRAYER SUGGESTION

➴ Spend some time in intercessory prayer. Hold each person lovingly in your mind while inviting Jesus to touch and heal. Pay attention to how Jesus reacts to each person, and pray that the Lord's response will become manifest. For example, if you perceive light around the person, pray that God's light will surround him or her.

If you are praying for victims of widespread devastation, such as an earthquake or war, try allowing yourself to feel some of the impact of the disaster. If you are willing to experience imaginatively some of the tragedy, you may find yourself at a loss for words. Don't worry. Just stay with your feelings and invite God to read the prayer of your heart. After a time of silence, thank God, and record your experience in your journal.

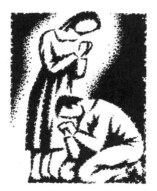

Reminder

For days I had been imagining over and over the final minutes inside the towers, and my consciousness was filled with screams, helplessness, and panic. This tape loop played constantly in my mind; and although I prayed about it, I could not move beyond the horror of it all.

A few days later I attended a meeting with my colleagues in Gestalt Pastoral Care Ecumenical Associates, and we prayed together as usual. In this small community, my prayer took on clearer focus. I prayed that God would enter into my "loop" and infuse it with grace without shutting my heart to the depth of the tragedy. I prayed to see the collapse of the towers through the eyes of resurrection.

Then I felt a shift that reminded me of the marvelous way Jesus spoke to me at the airport when my parents were killed. A conversation unwrapped itself between Jesus and me:

"Tilda, do you remember what I told you at the airport when your parents were killed?"

Jesus often asks me this question when I'm afraid.

"Yes, sure. You said, 'Don't be afraid. I'm always with you.'"

"Do you remember," Jesus responded, "how I helped you when you were so terrified right after the plane crash?"

Of course I remembered how I was marvelously sustained at age sixteen.

"Don't you think that I did the same for the people in the towers and on the planes? Don't you know I was there, offering each one just what he or she needed, just as I did for you? Don't you know that I was able to take away their fears, if they would let me, and welcome them home?"

With these gracious words I felt something change inside me. The screams I had been imagining didn't vanish, but they were overshadowed by a powerful awareness of God's love, which transcends suffering, fear, and death. A new image formed in my heart, an image as true as the horror, an image of hundreds of people being held and profoundly comforted as they died, an image of Jesus welcoming the people home.

PRAYER SUGGESTION

In your journal recall a time in your life of strong and luminous faith, a moment of God's unmistakable nearness. If you can't identify such a time, recall an important blessed event such as your marriage, the birth of a child, or recovery from a major illness. Describe the event in your journal in as much detail as you can remember. Go back in time and relive it. How was God present, and what did God communicate to you during that time?

Give thanks, and ask God to continue to remind you of that holy time. Allow it to impact you in the present. Put a symbol of it on your altar.

The Tears of Christ

RODNEY MILLER, a United Methodist pastor in Tamaqua, Pennsylvania, woke around 7:00 A.M. on September 11, two hours before the World Trade Center disaster began to unfold. Still drowsy, he began to pray even before he was fully awake. As he got out of bed he found himself sobbing uncontrollably, as if he was stricken with the deepest grief imaginable.

Rodney was bewildered. He couldn't think of anything that would cause him such profound sadness. The fact that crying does not come easily for Rodney added to his puzzlement. However, that morning tears and grief just seemed to come unbidden and mysteriously from some wellspring deep within. Finally he simply gave himself over to this strange occurrence, allowing his tears to flow until finished. Although he still had no idea why he cried, he felt an odd sense of rightness about it, and when the profusion of tears was over he felt better.

Later that day, Rodney was stunned and horrified as he watched the disaster on television. At the same time he felt an instant sense of recognition and peace that linked his inexplicable tears to the crashing planes and falling buildings. A certainty that he had been given a gift of profound mystery, that of crying the tears of Christ, enveloped him.

Rodney now believes that Christ embraced this new cross before it happened, that Jesus wept over New York just as he wept over Jerusalem. "As he came near and saw the city, he wept over it, saying, 'If you, even you, had only recognized on this day the things that make for peace! But now they are hidden from your eyes'" (Luke 19:41-42). Rodney believes that Jesus wept through him for all the people who would die and for those who would cause their deaths.

PRAYER SUGGESTION

🖙 This process invites you to surrender to God's work in you, even if that work is mysterious and contrary to your idea of how you should be healed. Find two pillows to bring to your prayer time; small throw pillows or bed pillows are fine. Each pillow represents a part of you.

Let one pillow symbolize the part of you that insists on your idea of how and when you need to be healed. Perhaps part of you clings to the idea that someone who has hurt you must apologize before you can let go of your pain, that a tragedy has to make sense before you will let God near, or that you must be healed physically right now.

Let the other pillow represent the part of you that has at least some measure of faith that God indeed wants to heal you—the part that willingly trusts God to heal you in the way God wants. Perhaps this side of you is tired of holding on to the past.

Sit on each pillow in turn, and speak as the part of you each pillow represents. Allow a conversation to develop between your two sides.

If you feel ready, surrender the "my agenda or nothing" pillow to Jesus, physically laying it before him. Hold the "faith" pillow in your arms.

How does Jesus react to your surrender? How do you feel? What has shifted inside? Thank God for what happened, and record your experience in your journal.

Silent Terrorism

UNITED CHURCH OF CHRIST pastor Norman C. Eddy has lived and worked in East Harlem for over fifty years. Always passionate about the church's need to work for justice and to alleviate suffering, Norm is now eighty-two and "retired." These days he coordinates a movement to improve public schools in East Harlem. An ecumenical prayer network supports the efforts of this community group. Bible study, prayer, and work for justice are always interwoven in the rich fabric of Norm's spirituality.

Before September 11 became a day that the world would remember, Norm rose early that Tuesday morning and began his plan to read the book of Isaiah straight through, all sixty-six chapters. A few hours later two verses from the first chapter flooded his consciousness. As the planes hit, Norm forcefully remembered having read:

> . . . your cities are burned with fire; in your very presence aliens devour your land. (Isaiah 1:7)

> Learn to do good; seek justice, rescue the oppressed, defend the orphan, plead for the widow. (1:17)

Norm says that his life is full of what he calls "divine

coincidences." He has encountered such epiphanies before in scripture. Even so, he was startled that Isaiah's words of twenty-seven hundred years ago would shimmer with such relevance today. Again the scripture challenged him to "learn to do good," to "seek justice," to "defend the orphan" and "plead for the widow," especially now that our city has been "burned with fire." Now, more than ever, he is aware of what he calls "silent terrorism"—the terrorism of substandard education and inadequate housing, the terrorism of poverty and racism, the shattering of families. He knows that silent terrorism will worsen in the days ahead. Just two months after the America's war on terrorism began, $3.4 million had been cut from the budget of School District No. 4 and its already struggling twenty-two public schools in East Harlem.

Norm feels that we are in an extremely critical time in human history. He knows that since September 11 a new quality of fervent prayer is going up all over the world. The wind of the Holy Spirit seems to be blowing strongly. At the same time, demonic spirits rage, seeking to destroy. This cosmic battle calls all of us to renewed faith and commitment to live the gospel so that all of God's children have a share in the world's resources.

PRAYER SUGGESTION

❧ Prayerfully listen to God's voice in your heart as you write examples of silent terrorism in your journal. Think about your own lifestyle. Does it contribute to silent terrorism? Let this awareness generate confession and prayer for the victims of silent terrorism.

In silence, listen for any invitation God extends for you to become involved in erasing silent terrorism in your community. Record your discernment in your journal.

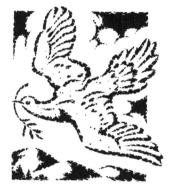

"He Descended into Hell . . ."

Everett Wabst, a most unusual Baptist minister, was a New York City firefighter for twenty-seven years. Ordained in 1982 while still a firefighter, he served as an informal chaplain to the fire department until 1999 when he retired and became an "honorary fire chaplain." Although the fire department usually hires chaplains, Everett's job is voluntary. He does it because he loves to serve in this way and feels called to this ministry. He had no idea that in the fall of 2001 his unique background would be exactly what was needed to minister to the hundreds of rescue and recovery workers at ground zero.

After September 11, Everett's expertise as a firefighter allowed him to go places no other member of the clergy could reach. One day after the attack he found himself deep in the wreckage with a crew of firefighters. They had climbed up precarious piles, traversed deep canyons on ladders hastily thrown across shifting piles of rubble, and had clambered up inside a mountain of smoldering wreckage. All of them knew that the giant girders scattered above them could shift at any time. They had no guarantees that any of them would make it out alive. Yet they stayed more than twenty hours to dig out some dozen bodies.

As each body was discovered and unearthed, the firefighters stopped for prayer, with Everett blessing the body. In that literal hellhole the perpetrators were not cursed, even though the workers knew that the bodies they carried out might belong to people they knew personally. Instead a sense of prayer, blessing, and God's presence prevailed. Everett was moved that each body was treated as a precious treasure, lovingly cradled in the arms of the recovery team.

That day the recovery workers faced the fact that some bodies were so vaporized by the intense heat that they would never be recovered. They agreed that the thick air filling their lungs contained "the blood of the saints." Where there could easily have been undiluted despair and horror, there was also a sense of holiness.

The liturgical stole Everett wore that day is now unspeakably grimy, but he will never wash it. For him this stole is a healing icon. It reminds him of God's faithful presence even in the face of unimaginable evil.

Every so often a man would grab Everett and hug him, thanking him for being there. Everett insists the gratitude was not about him personally; it really belonged to God who was transforming the horror into something new. Everett believes that "evil won a round" with the attack, but almost immediately "the Lord started turning things around."

PRAYER SUGGESTION

☙ Pray the following psalm aloud, pausing often to connect the psalmist's experience with your own.

Where can I go from your spirit?
Or where can I flee from your presence?
If I ascend to heaven, you are there;
if I make my bed in Sheol, you are there.
If I take the wings of the morning
and settle at the farthest limits of the sea,
even there your hand shall lead me,
and your right hand shall hold me fast.
If I say, "Surely the darkness shall cover me,
and the light around me become night,"
even the darkness is not dark to you;
the night is as bright as the day,
for darkness is as light to you. (Psalm 139:7-12)

In your journal, paraphrase this psalm, drawing from your own darkest times or from 9/11 images that haunt you. Even if your present emotions suggest otherwise, let yourself cling to faith in God's presence. For example:

If someone I love dies, if a good friend betrays me, if my parents abused me, if I have done something terrible, if I am in a place of hell where love seems to have vanished, even if you, God, seem to have abandoned me, you are still present. No matter what happens, no matter where I go, I can't get away from your loving presence. . . .

Mention all the details of your suffering that occur to you. Affirm God's steadfast love in all of it.

What did you discover as you wrote your psalm? Try praying your psalm daily for a while, and see what happens.

Hard Questions

Reverend Everett Wabst, the ex-firefighter turned fire department chaplain, was called to ground zero on September 11. Since then he has witnessed countless miracles as God works to bring good out of evil.

One of the first miracles Everett recognized was the surprisingly high number of people who escaped death. Many commentators have pondered the large numbers of people who were late to work that day for various reasons or didn't go to work at all. Countless people returned home for a forgotten item, were delayed in the subway, or made a rare stop for coffee that particular morning. Many people, Everett among them, believe that God greatly limited the number of people who would die that day by a cluster of miraculous delays and diversions. A group of about one hundred World Trade Center workers, for example, was on Staten Island the morning of September 11, attending the funeral of a colleague. The priest told them that the timing of their colleague's death from cancer probably saved their lives. Such stories abound.

Everett also reports that when the towers were bombed in 1993, it took several hours for everyone to stream out of the buildings. Following that attack, the fire department mapped the escape routes of the towers and calculated the number of people who could walk down the stairs and out of the towers in a given time. By these fire department calculations, at least 20,000 people should have died on September 11. Instead, about 3,000 people perished. While 3,000 is a number that tears at the heart, it is surprisingly small in comparison to what might have been. Fire department experts are at a loss to explain this relatively small number of deaths that radically differs from what might have been expected.

Reflecting this bewilderment, officials estimate now that perhaps 25,000 people were in the towers on the morning of the attacks instead of the usual 50,000 during business hours. Experts say this estimate is very low. However, even assuming the accuracy of this low figure Everett says it was physically impossible that all but 3,000 people could have walked down the stairs to safety in the time between the attacks and the collapse of the buildings. He and others have had to conclude that somehow God helped a lot of people to safety that day. There have been countless heartfelt prayers of thanksgiving since September 11 for God's miraculous deliverance from death.

This is small comfort to the families of the 3,000 who died. Naturally they ask why God would deliver some but not others. Why their husband, wife, son, daughter, sister, brother? Others ask, Why didn't God simply stop the hijackers? If God could make hundreds of people late to work, surely God could have foiled the plans of nineteen terrorists.

These questions shouldn't prompt easy answers. When evil grasps hold of human freedom, it is especially difficult to make sense of senseless killing. Throughout history faithful Christians have struggled to understand the problem of theodicy—why terrible things happen to innocent people. Even theologians have trouble finding explanations. Glib replies to such anguished questions dishonor both the deep suffering of family members and the mystery of God's being.

Even though human understanding is too small to explain why God didn't act differently, we can still respond to the questions with faith. We can ask for grace to believe that God loves us even in our most terrible circumstances: in disaster and fear, in despair and grief, and in our deepest suffering. Even as we recognize that evil exists, we can pray for eyes of faith to see how God is working to heal and to make all things new. We can pray our hardest questions, asking God to show us answers that will make it possible for us to go on. We can open ourselves to God's response to our questions, knowing that God's reply may be surprising and different for different persons. Perhaps we can begin to affirm that miracles come in many different guises: miracles of deliverance, miracles of reconciliation, miracles of healing, miracles of peace that passes understanding, miracles of evil contained, and most certainly miracles of resurrection.

One day early in the rescue operations, Everett Wabst climbed the mountain of debris to a place where he could see the entire carnage of the towers. Although he fully realized the horror of this scene of mass destruction, his attention was captured by the thousands of workers swarming over the wreckage. He saw them risking their lives to dig by hand into the rubble. He witnessed their passionate dedication to saving any lives they could. He saw this and gave thanks—thanks for the many good people to whom God gave courage; thanks for his background as a firefighter that allowed him to help at a crucial time; and thanks for God's loving, healing presence permeating the site.

Everett Wabst has eyes of faith.

PRAYER SUGGESTION

➽ What are your hardest questions? List them in your journal in their sharpest form. You don't need to protect God from your true feelings, nor do you need to soften the terrible questions that can keep you awake at night.

Now try reframing your questions along the lines suggested under "Beginning the Journey of Healing" on page 29, changing "why?" into "how?" or "what?" How do you feel when you ask your questions this way? See if you are ready to invite the Holy Spirit to answer you in God's way and in God's time. Decide whether you will pray for an answer that satisfies your heart.

As you feel led, enter into a faith-imagination process with a newly framed question. Wait in silence for God to work in you. Even if your faith-imagination prayer does not yield a complete answer, write it down anyway. Know that your answer may take time and will probably come together only after many different prayer experiences. Don't give up. Keep asking, listening, and writing whatever God gives in your journal. As you keep the questions open, expect an answer to emerge.

Holy Ground (Zero)

A FEW DAYS before Christmas in 2001, I went to ground zero with fire department chaplain Everett Wabst. The gray air was acrid with smoke and the stench of still-smoldering fire. Many people wore masks but coughed nonetheless. As Everett and I descended into the deep hole of wreckage, we walked on shifting shards of twisted metal and fine gray ash. Almost nothing was recognizable—not a computer, a desk, or a piece of glass. Huge girders, bent and folded, were thrown about like twigs. Unaccountably a perfectly intact pair of polka-dot boxer shorts, complete with store tag, was embedded in a mound of rubble. Huge earth-moving machines rumbled nearby, shaking the unstable ground on which we stood.

The grimy men working in the pit clearly welcomed Everett's presence. Many of them stopped their work to speak to him for a few minutes. Some men had been working here since the disaster; others had been conscripted for just a few days. No one could forget that the group was working in a mass grave and that the ashes under their feet quite possibly held human remains. Everett knew they wanted to be reminded that God was here and that this pit was holy ground.

At one point, however, the workers needed no reminding. A huge shovel unearthed a fire helmet; all work stopped immediately. As the enormous shovel backed away, men came from all corners of the sixteen-acre site carrying small garden tools: little shovels and rakes, tiny scoops and trowels. With remarkable tenderness these burly men dug by hand for any other shred of clothing or part of a body.

As Everett and I waited nearby, I spoke with a man who had been a firefighter all his life. Following family tradition, his son had also become a firefighter and had perished in the disaster. The father, now retired, had come here every day until they located the body of his son. Now he was volunteering "to help other people find their sons and wives and daughters." Although he did not speak of God, surely God had empowered him to turn the still fresh anguish of his personal tragedy into an opportunity to serve others.

The men digging by hand found very little. They discovered a fragment of human tissue that they carefully placed in a container for identification. Mingled with fatigue, disappointment, and numbness was an attitude of profound respect and holiness.

Everett says that being in the pit at ground zero humbles him. He counts it a rare privilege to bless bodies and body parts as they are lovingly unearthed. Whenever a body or a body part is discovered, the workers insist on calling clergy over for prayer and blessing. For a few moments everything stops as weary men join hands and pray for the dead person and his or her family. Both Everett and I were deeply moved by the profound respect these exhausted recovery workers, themselves traumatized, have shown for human life. Even in the face of a horrifying job, they have not forgotten the truth that these were human beings, known and loved by God.

PRAYER SUGGESTION

Ask Jesus to take you on a visit to ground zero. If he is willing to do this, go with him in your imagination. Walk slowly. Look around you. Talk to people you meet. Feel your emotions, and tell Jesus how you feel. Are you horrified? afraid? angry? How does your body react? If you feel tearful, let yourself weep for the people who died in the towers. As much as you are able, take in exactly what happened here, and share it with Jesus.

At the same time, remain aware of the way Jesus frames your experience. Ask him to show you how this site is holy ground. Ask him any other questions you might have. How does he shape your attention? What does he say? Does he touch you? If so, what does his touching communicate to you? How do you react? Do you want to hold his hand or bury your face in his chest?

Thank Jesus, and walk away from the site before ending your prayer. In your journal, record what Jesus taught you at ground zero.

Surprise

ON 9/11, the Reverend Molly O'Neill Louden, a psychotherapist and an Episcopal priest in Connecticut, went to visit her former teacher and training supervisor. Although she does not share Molly's Christian faith, this woman has been an important mentor to Molly.

Molly describes her teacher's spirituality as a mixture of "Russian Orthodox/Jewish/Buddhist/Native American." Her teacher often seeks the help of "spirit guides" as she invokes certain animals or other entities through various meditation techniques.

On the day of the disaster, this woman told Molly she had searched for a spirit guide to help shape her response to the tragedy. To her utter surprise, she experienced Jesus speaking words into her heart about the people who perished.

Molly's teacher reported that Jesus said to her, "Not one of them is lost. I have every one of them. I'll be gathering more this afternoon and evening, but know that not one of them is lost."

PRAYER SUGGESTION

❧ Gift wrap a small box and put it where you can see it often. Let it serve as a reminder that God's work is often surprising and always a gift. Each time you see it, thank God and open yourself to the possibility that God may have a surprise in store for you.

Write about God's surprises in your journal.

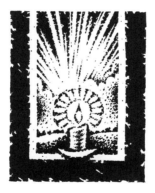

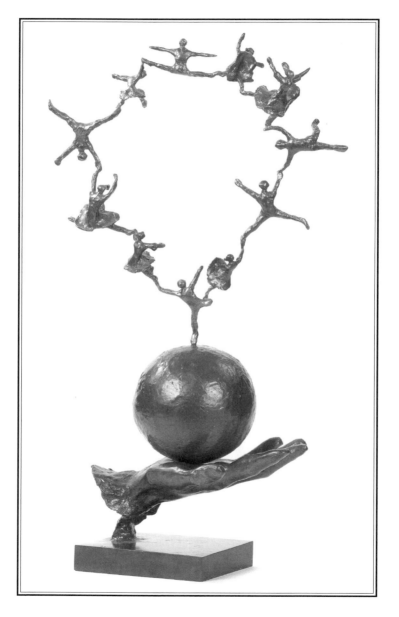

HE HAS THE WHOLE WORLD IN HIS HANDS

The Whole World

WHEN THE PLANES crashed on September 11, the Reverend Wanda M. Lundy, a Presbyterian pastor in Edgewater, New Jersey, was two months pregnant. Her first thought was for her unborn child and the chaotic world her child would inherit. She wept a lot that day, and her anguished lament for her child was, "Why can't we just get along? Why does it have to be this way?"

Although deeply sympathetic to those who suffered and died in the attacks, Wanda was astonished at how Americans reacted to the disaster as if nothing like this had ever happened before. She recognizes that terrorism happens all over the world, even if we Americans manage to ignore most of it. She emphatically points out that September 11 was not the only time people in this country died from terrorism. As a woman of African-American and Native American heritage, she is keenly conscious that American history is bloodied by the horrors of slavery and the cruel and shameful treatment of native peoples.

Wanda believes that pain and suffering provide the context for growing closer to our Creator. Oppressed people simply have to "lean on the Lord." Deep suffering gives birth to the conviction that God has the victory.

Wanda prays that out of our suffering as a nation since September 2001 will come a new commitment to peace and justice for all people and an expansion of our definition of *family* to include the whole world. She fervently hopes we will learn to trust God more fully and respond to others more faithfully. "If we allow this disaster to pass without changing us," she contends, "the people who died on 9/11 will have died in vain."

PRAYER SUGGESTION

🐟 Bring a map of the world to your place of prayer. Let your eyes travel over the map until you stop at the name of a city outside the United States. Read aloud the name, and pause for a moment. If you know even one of the issues facing the people of that city or about how the people in that city might be suffering, pray specifically for the people there. If you don't know much about the city, pray that God will heal and bless the inhabitants. Repeat this prayer for other places on the map.

Record your experience in your journal. Resolve to find out more about the cities for which you prayed. Pay particular attention to news accounts about them, and let the news prompt you to continue your prayers.

Rage in Church

JUDITH, a United Methodist pastor in Ohio, opened the church for prayer and sharing on September 11. That evening people gathered, hungry for comfort and for a place to acknowledge the jumble of intense emotions engulfing them. Judith invited members of the congregation to bring to the Lord whatever they were feeling, assuring them that God would meet them in their depths.

One young man, a member of the church, took Judith's words to heart. Bursting with fury, he began to rage at the attackers. He yelled. He ranted. He spewed hatred for terrorists. He insisted that the United States should immediately bomb the hell out of Afghanistan.

The young man's anger blew itself out finally, and he sat down spent and sweaty. Wisely, Judith did not lecture him about love and forgiveness. Instead, she said how glad she was that he felt free enough in God's house to express exactly what was inside him. The congregation, unaccustomed to such raw emotion in church, was a little frightened by it. But Judith's permission-giving words enabled members to receive his volatile statements without overt judgment. In fact, this congregation, which had always found it difficult to share personally when asked for prayer concerns, suddenly found itself praying together. In particular the church members gave thanks that this young man felt free to share his anger with them.

After the service the young man hung around to speak to Judith privately. Although a little embarrassed by his emotional display, he really wanted to tell her that his anger was gone. No longer did he obsess about vengeance or feel hatred. Instead, he had discovered that allowing himself to erupt so deeply paved the way for a major healing. The church's acceptance of him even after witnessing his poisonous rage moved him, and the new peace and sense of freedom seeping into his heart utterly surprised him.

PRAYER SUGGESTION

❧ This prayer suggestion invites you to express in depth before God the anger you may harbor inside. Remember that anger is a healthy response that leads to healing and forgiveness—if you don't hold onto it. What you are about to do will hurt no one. Expressing anger this way is a form of confession in which you own up to what is inside you. If you are frightened to show anger, you may need a therapist experienced in physical release of emotions to help you. If, however, you feel comfortable, go ahead. You will need large markers or crayons, large pieces of paper, a plastic bat, and some old pillows.

Ask Jesus to be with you and to help you express whatever anger is inside so you can let go of it. On a large sheet of paper, write what angers you. Write it large! Scribble it fast! For example:

Being told I'm stupid makes me FURIOUS!

How dare she hurt me!

Terrorists!

I hate _____!

Let your body express your anger by hitting the pillows with the bat. Yell! Growl! Stomp! Go as far as you want with this. If you are really angry, don't stop with one or two swats of the bat. Allow your body the time and energy to discover and release your anger in all its intensity.

How do you feel afterward? Does your body feel more roomy? less tense? What has happened to your anger? What else is true about you right now? How is Jesus responding to you? Ask him to transform the anger you have released into energy for healing. Thank God for your experience, and record it in your journal.

A Call to Repentance

RHODA GLICK, a psychotherapist and student at Eastern Mennonite Seminary in Harrisonburg, Virginia, is known for her upbeat personality and her mature, vibrant faith. Rhoda was worshiping in the seminary chapel when someone announced that the World Trade towers in New York City had been hit by two hijacked planes piloted by terrorists.

After the service many students remained in the chapel, Rhoda among them. As she prayed there, Rhoda had an experience that went far beyond her usual psychotherapeutic focus on personal dynamics. To her surprise, she found herself gripped with a profound sense of the need for national repentance. She became acutely aware of the disparity of wealth and resources between the United States and the rest of the world. She felt in her body our greed, possessiveness, self-involvement, and lust for power. She was reminded of how easy it is to confuse following Christ with patriotism.

As clear as the need for repentance was to Rhoda, she felt certain that the disaster was not God's punishment. God did not send this tragedy to teach a lesson, nor did God want it to happen. Instead, God was using the tragedy to offer the healing that follows deep confession. A scripture passage floated to her awareness: "If my people who are called by my name humble themselves, pray, seek my face, and turn from their wicked ways, then I will hear from heaven, and will forgive their sin and heal their land" (2 Chron. 7:14).

Thus Rhoda felt a call to repent, not just for herself, but for the whole world, especially on behalf of those who don't know to repent for themselves. "We can confess sin for those who don't know how to do it," she said, "because we participate in communal sin as members of the human race."

It was not just the need for repentance, however, that flooded Rhoda's spirit. She also sensed a call to follow Christ more truly, to participate in the healing God intends for us as a nation and as world citizens. "God's redemptive work," she said, "makes the tragedy a unique opportunity for the human family to learn to live together in a new way, characterized by sharing and tolerance and mutual respect. We need to remember that even now God is making all things new."

Prayer Suggestion

🖎 Take to heart Rhoda's passion for national repentance. In the Hebrew Bible, the priests often prayed on behalf of the entire community of Israelites. Let a priestly prayer of confession and intercession take shape in your heart. As you pray, write in your journal.

See if you can involve others in such a prayer. Call a friend or two and get together for an evening. Perhaps a more permanent group will grow out of it.

Can you help organize a service of confession and recommitment at your church?

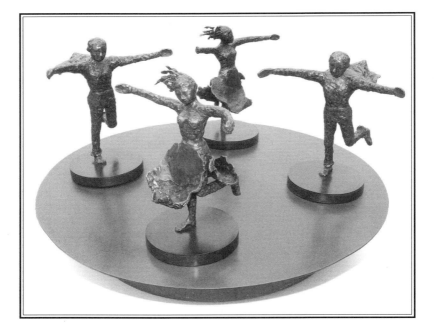

FORGIVENESS

Forgiveness

⌒

DR. ROSE GAUHAR, a pediatrician and member of Linden Heights United Methodist Church in Parkville, Maryland, came to the United States in 1976 from Quetta, Pakistan. Quetta, a town on the border of Pakistan and Afghanistan, has been the scene of much turmoil since September 11.

Rose brought to this country her Christian faith, her medical degree, and a desire to begin a new life. She also brought what she calls "a lot of garbage": prejudice, anger, and near-hatred for Muslim extremists. Christians are a small, persecuted minority in Pakistan, and her family and close friends suffered greatly. Although she had some good Muslim friends in Pakistan, Rose's anger toward Muslim extremists had smoldered inside her for years.

The military action in Afghanistan following the September 11 disaster brought her seething anger to the surface. She remembers watching television footage of wounded and dying Afghans and thinking despite herself, *Oh, good, another one down.* A committed Christian, Rose was horrified at the extent of the vengeance inside her. "I was an awful, ugly person until God healed me," she reflects.

One Sunday in October 2001, Rose felt unwell and decided to pray at home instead of going to church. She remembers sitting by a window that morning reading a passage from Ephesians about God's love.

> For this reason I bow my knees before the Father, from whom every family in heaven and on earth takes its name. I pray that, according to the riches of his glory, he may grant that you may be strengthened in your inner being with power through his Spirit, and that Christ may dwell in your hearts through faith, as you are being rooted and grounded in love. I pray that you may have the power to comprehend, with all the saints, what is the breadth and length and height and depth, and to know the love of Christ that surpasses knowledge, so that you may be filled with all the fullness of God. (3:14-19)

Upon reading these words, Rose had what she calls a "heart experience, a flooding of the love of God for me and for the Muslims; this love was cleansing, and I was engulfed in it." She came to see that God feels sorrow for the destructive actions on both sides. A new song in her heart told her that Muslims are as much God's children as Christians. That morning she no longer had a sense of "me here and them there." Rather, she affirmed, "We all need God's love." This realization was accompanied by an image of the cross absorbing her inner darkness. The healing love of God flowed out of the cross, finding a new place in her heart and helping her bloom. "I'm a flower that is rooted and grounded in the love of Christ, who is everything to me," she said. "He filled me with cleansing love and removed the hatred."

This experience, as marvelous as it was, did not take hold instantly. Occasionally the old anger surges up, and as she says, "I must double up my prayers. I see that this is who I am without God, and I can still be quite hawkish. But God is changing me as I ask for more healing."

Rose feels a special urgency to pray for Muslims these days. "I'm just so sad that some of them are so misled," she says. "Tying bombs to their shoes, hitting buildings with planes to blast themselves into paradise—these are such tragic actions. I just pray that we can all eat at the same table someday." For herself she prays that she "may have the power to comprehend with all the saints what is the breadth and length and height and depth, and to know the love of Christ that surpasses knowledge" (Eph. 3:18).

PRAYER SUGGESTION

🌀 When there has been deep hurt, genuine healing includes forgiveness of the one who hurt you. Knowing this, many Christians lock the depth of their rage in their bodies while smiling with immediate words of forgiveness. Although they are trying to be faithful, they try to forgive much too quickly, before they have had time to do the necessary inner work of real forgiveness. Especially in cases of deep wounding, forgiveness is a process that takes time and a good measure of God's grace.

Admitting the depth of your anger is the first step in forgiving. Sit quietly with your journal for a time to center yourself, asking Jesus to shine the light of truth in you. Ask yourself these questions:

Am I holding onto a grudge?
Am I holding out for revenge or an apology?
Am I holding in the expression of my anger?

If you have not already found a way to express the depth of your anger, explore ways to let it go physically. Don't skip over this part of the process! You might start with the prayer suggestion on pages 152–53. A Gestalt or Bioenergetic therapist can be helpful at this stage.

Once you have gone to the bottom of your anger, honestly ask yourself what you are gaining from holding onto it. Does being angry help you feel powerful? Does your grudge somehow punish the one who hurt you? Does your demand for an apology keep things familiar and you comfortable? If even a small part of you is not yet ready to change, admit it before God and write it in your journal.

Are you ready now to ask God to prepare you to offer forgiveness? Or are you ready to be ready? Let your prayer be honest as you ask God to prepare your heart for real forgiveness. Even when most of you is willing to forgive, there is still a good chance you can't quite do it emotionally. God, however, can bring you there. Ask the Holy Spirit to do the work of forgiveness in you, letting the love of Christ flow through you. When you have done all you can, depend on God for the rest.

Stay with your process of forgiveness for as long as it takes. Keep track of how the Holy Spirit heals you, and thank God for your progress at each step.

Meeting God Face-to-Face

ONE AFTERNOON a few weeks before the disaster, Wanda Windsor, pastor of Evergreen United Methodist Church in Fort Bragg, California, spent time with the children in the church's after-school program, a ministry to special children. Some kids in the program are hearing or sight impaired; others from foreign countries have been adopted by American families in Fort Bragg. Most feel their differences from other children both at school and in the community.

On this particular afternoon, the children chattered and worked on crafts as usual when a visitor, a man traveling on a bicycle, interrupted their routine. Seeing his fatigue, Wanda let him in; and soon curious kids surrounded him. The man was trying to get home to San Francisco, but bad luck had plagued him, and he was running out of money. On impulse he had stopped by the church, wondering if the church might have a food pantry.

The church happened to have a good deal of food left over from a funeral luncheon earlier that day. Raiding the refrigerator, the children set out a meal for the hungry man and sacked up more leftovers for him to take on the road. The kids also pooled their resources and gave him a little money. Then they did what was utterly natural in their church:

They surrounded the man and prayed for his safe journey.

A week after the September 11 disaster, the man called Wanda to say that he had made it to San Francisco. Profoundly shaken by the terrible events, he felt moved to call and say thanks. The tragedy had prompted him to think seriously about his life, and the Fort Bragg kids had come forcefully to mind. As a result, he had resolved to help other strangers as he had been helped by the children. He told Wanda, "Tell your children I met God face-to-face at your church. I just want them to know how much it meant to me."

But not only the stranger on a bike was changed by this grace-filled encounter. The kids in the program, well-acquainted with both rejection and kindness from others, had seldom experienced the joy of helping someone truly in need. Exhilarated and empowered, they were delighted to know they had made a difference in this man's life.

Wanda shared the children's experience in a sermon that began with a story about a sparrow holding up the sky with his tiny, spindly legs. The little bird explained that he was "doing what he could to help."

Now the kids in Evergreen's after-school care program enthusiastically collect money in a jar labeled "sparrow change." They want to be ready in case another tired and hungry stranger comes to the church door.

PRAYER SUGGESTION

🐦 In your journal, write eight to ten sentences beginning with "I'm just . . ." and ending with "to make a difference." Here are some examples:

"I'm just too old to make a difference."

"I'm just one person, so I can't make a difference."

"I'm just too messed up to make a difference."

"I'm just not well-educated, so I can't make a difference."

"I'm just an egghead scholar, so how can I make a difference?"

"I'm just too busy to make a difference."

The idea of this exercise is to explore the deeply ingrained "tapes" that play in your mind. Even if you know better, messages like these can powerfully shape your behavior.

Now, as best you can, surrender your list to the Lord. You may want to put the written list on your altar or imagine giving it to Jesus. Stay aware of your feelings as you make this surrender. Ask that the real truth be written on your heart, and that you might have the eyes of faith to see Christ in the face of a stranger who may need your help.

Each night put some "sparrow change" in a jar. As the jar fills, be alert to needs that present themselves to you. Watch your mail. Scan the newspaper. Prayerfully decide where your sparrow change will do the most good. When your jar is full, give the money away.

A Muslim Speaks

TRAVIS JACKSON, a Sufi Muslim and a student of Sheikh Tosun Efendi of Turkey, is a prisoner at Arthur Kill Correctional Facility on Staten Island. Before I met him, several inmates insisted that he was "the smartest guy in the whole prison." After talking to Mr. Jackson for just a few minutes I am inclined to believe them. He is articulate, well-informed, and speaks with a direct gaze and gentle smile. He is also a man of devout prayer and faithful hope.

"It was a horrific act," he said of the 9/11 disaster, "and inconsistent with the mainstream beliefs of Islam. We have our fanatic fundamentalists, just as Christians do." He explained that Islamic fundamentalists focus on the literal meaning of the Koran while ignoring the essence of Islam found in the written traditions of the prophet Muhammad. A large collection of sayings, teachings, and stories from Muhammad's life instructs followers never to "slay non-combatants," especially women and children. These traditions, called "hadiths," also admonish followers not to wantonly kill animals. Nor should they cut trees or burn grass without good reason.

Travis Jackson describes his first reaction, upon hearing the news of the 9/11 attack, as "selfish." He greatly feared what the actions of a few Muslims might mean for Muslims everywhere. He remembers thinking, *Here we go again. Now we'll all be targets.* He knew all too well the possibility of suspicion, prejudice, and worse being visited upon the Muslim community.

Travis's second reaction came close on the heels of the first. As grief for the tragedy washed over him, he knew that he had to pray for the victims and their families. He did not discriminate in his prayer; he included "whites, blacks, Muslims, Christians, Jews, everybody."

Five months after the disaster Travis spoke of the hope growing inside him. "Maybe out of this tragedy can come healing," he said. "Maybe even some interfaith dialogue."

Travis Jackson's hope for interfaith dialogue may be coming true, at least a little. Many neighborhood interfaith educational programs have popped up all over New York City. For instance, in February 2002 an important conference on Christian-Muslim dialogue, sponsored by the Metropolitan-Duane United Methodist Church in Manhattan and the Methodist Federation for Social Action, took place at the Church Center at the United Nations. About thirty United Methodist clergy and laypersons attended the daylong event. One enthusiastic participant reported, "This seminar laid the groundwork for Christian-Muslim dialogue in the future. It helped cultivate a new sensitivity to Islam and the political and religious realities in the Afghan region. And, personally, I learned a lot about Islam I didn't know."

PRAYER SUGGESTION

☞ As you search your heart, ask the Holy Spirit to reveal the truth to you about your own hatred and mistrust. Ask yourself these questions:

What person or group do I hate?

What groups do I automatically mistrust?

Which groups scare me?

Honestly confess your feelings in your journal. Honesty about your true feelings is the first step toward healing.

Know that you cannot change how you feel just by wanting to. You may have a good personal reason for being angry or scared. As a Christian, however, you are called to root out any trait that is not Christlike and to pray for God to heal you.

Another important step in this healing is to pray for your "enemies," just as Travis Jackson did when he prayed for everyone, including some who might persecute Muslims. Without discounting your anger or fear (which may still be there), try praying for your enemies. Pray for your betrayer, your abuser, the one who caused you pain. Pray for those you consider to be political enemies.

What happened to you as you prayed? How have your feelings changed or perhaps shifted?

Record your experience in your journal.

Crying for the World

Dr. George McClain, a member of the Doctor of Ministry faculty at New York Theological Seminary, served for twenty-five years as the executive director of the Methodist Federation for Social Action. Since he is also my husband, he willingly shared his faith experience related to the 9/11 disaster.

For days after September 11, when not actually weeping, George was close to tears. He remembers flying to Indiana ten days after the attacks and, rather astonished at himself, sobbing uncontrollably from Newark to Cleveland. He cried for the people who suffered and died and for their families. He cried for New York City, which had been his home for forty years.

During this tumultuous time George also felt an intense sense of identification with strangers on the subway and street, deeply aware of his common vulnerability with them. Knowing that a traumatic experience linked them provided a new connection and made him acutely aware that everyone he met was "made in the image of God and was being sustained by God."

At the same time, a sense of isolation quickly set in. George felt like much of his culture had suddenly become supernationalistic, and, in many cases, vengeful. While most people were displaying American flags, George, feeling the need to remember the entire human community, searched in vain for a whole earth flag that displays a picture of the earth from the moon. In contrast to the prevailing winds, George remained convinced the disaster was not just an attack on the United States but on all humanity. He points out that not only were hundreds of foreigners killed in those buildings, but anguished cries were raised all over the globe. In the forty-eight hours after the attack, George received phone calls from friends and family around the world. Swiss cousins in particular reported that all of Switzerland had closed down in shock and mourning.

George became aware of how seductive the false god of nationalism can be and how challenging it is to stay focused on the teachings of Jesus, especially when we feel our security threatened. For him, the biblical response to disaster includes soul searching and repentance for any national sins that may have contributed to underlying factors. He fervently prays and works for peace—a genuine, worldwide peace that embraces the entire human family.

George's concern is not only global. He is dean of a program offered by the New York Theological Seminary at Arthur Kill Correctional Facility. Inmate graduates from this yearlong program had clamored for a second-year class in the fall of 2001, but he couldn't figure out what the course would be or who would teach it. But after September 11, he felt a call from God to teach a course himself on the history of New York City, as "my own way of expressing my love for my adopted city." He was delighted when our daughter, Shana Norberg-McClain, decided to teach along with him.

The class helped inmates, mostly New Yorkers whose experience of the city had largely been confined to their neighborhoods, become appreciative citizens of their own city to which they would return eventually. It was a moving experience for George and Shana to join the men in exploring both New York's often shameful treatment of minorities, as well as its amazing diversity, rich cultural gifts, and prominent role in struggles for justice.

For the following several months George's tears remained mostly beneath the surface. But then one afternoon, triggered by a story about civil rights martyrs, as well as a photo mosaic of September 11 victims, a new flood of tears cascaded through him. He cried for the injustice, violence, and raw evil that permeates our world. He cried for people who died in the civil rights movement of the 1960s, in which he had been heavily involved. He cried for the wasted lives of the inmates he was teaching and for the immense struggles they would face to reintegrate into society after years of incarceration. He cried for all the people, past and present, who have experienced cruel acts of war.

This time his tears seemed to have a clear meaning. Although his emotions were certainly involved, he sensed that his tears were much more than a personal emotional release. The uncontrolled, prolonged weeping had become a work of prayer, and he felt God's own tears being shed through him—a surprising answer to his prayer, taken from the prayer attributed to Saint Francis: "O Lord, make me an instrument of your peace."

PRAYER SUGGESTION

❧ John 11:28-44 recounts how Jesus cried with Mary, Lazarus's sister, when Lazarus died. Jesus must have cried long and hard to merit mention in John's Gospel.

Let yourself imaginatively travel back in time to the Galilee of two thousand years ago. Join Jesus and Mary as they grieve for Lazarus. Can you see them? Do you hear their sobs and wailing? Can you feel their sorrow?

In your imagination let the rest of the story unfold as Jesus calls Lazarus out of his tomb. Let yourself experience the shock, the incredulity, and the joy of friends and relatives as Lazarus is set free from his grave clothes. Can you hear them shrieking with excitement? Do you see them drop to their knees in awe? How does this story play out in your prayerful imagination?

Now invite Jesus, Mary, and Lazarus to come with you to your own place and time of sorrow. Pay attention to what they do and say. Do they weep with you? Do they give comfort? How do you experience them?

Ask Jesus to show you how in your own story he is bringing forth life out of the tomb. Wait in silence and expectancy for Jesus to act.

Continue praying for resurrection in your life. As it occurs, give thanks and record it in your journal.

"I'm Calling Them"

Lois Pongó is a massage therapist in Oyster Bay, New York. She was busy in the months following the World Trade Center disaster, frequently seeing people with physical responses to the events of September 11. She described the physical reactions of tension and fear as "ossified horror." It was profoundly draining for her to so often put her hands on this embodied devastation.

On the other hand, Lois saw that people were much more ready to talk about their pain after 9/11. "The crust, the shell has been ripped away," she said, "and now everyone seems more able to cry and to say what they really feel." She feels good about this new openness, but it too has contributed to the intensity of her work.

About three weeks after the disaster Lois went to a healing service at Parsippany United Methodist Church in Parsippany, New Jersey. Feeling exhausted and weighed down by all that she had felt from others, as well as her own reaction to the tragedy, she needed healing herself. What emerged uppermost in her consciousness was the devastation of those grieving the death of spouses. When the time came for laying on of hands, she asked for prayer for the husbands and wives who lost life partners in the inferno.

As hands were laid on Lois, prayers were offered that God would comfort the bereaved widows and widowers and give them the peace that passes all understanding. During the prayer, Lois sensed God speaking to her. "I'm calling them. I'm calling them. I'm calling them," she heard with her ears of faith.

These simple but immensely reassuring words lifted Lois's fatigue and gave her new hope. Her experience reminded her that God attends to everybody, giving comfort and faith, calling each person into an experience of God's presence. "Jesus is standing at the door, knocking, and people are responding. God is in charge of their healing, not me," she said with relief. Clearly God also was in charge of Lois's healing that night, giving her exactly the words she needed.

PRAYER SUGGESTION

✠ Ask prayerfully if you have taken on anyone (besides a child) as your responsibility. Do you feel responsible for a friend or family member's happiness? Does any part of you believe that it is up to you to bring someone from confusion to clarity or from depression to cheerfulness? Is it somehow up to you to make up for the childhood sufferings of your parents? Is there anyone you are trying to fix or wish you could fix? In other words, in what ways do you try to take on God's job?

Feel the physical heaviness of these impossible assignments. Where in your body do you carry these people? Your neck? Your shoulders? Your chest? What is this burden doing to you physically?

Remembering that Jesus, not you, is the Savior and healer, surrender these people to God's care and healing. Notice how you feel after your prayer. Does your body feel looser? If not, consider getting a professional massage. Continue your surrendering prayer as the massage therapist works. Record your experience in your journal.

In the following days, continue to pray for the persons whose concerns you used to carry, but use your journal to keep surrendering your false responsibility to heal them. Continue to thank God for taking your burden.

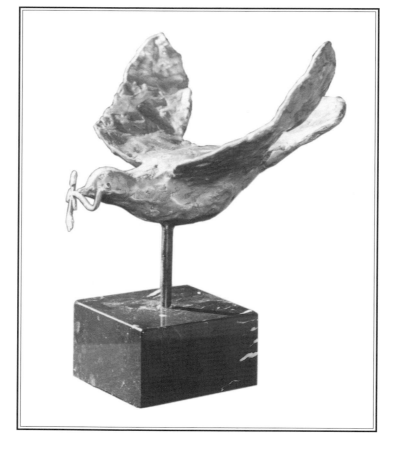

DOVE OF PEACE

Loving Our Enemies

WALTER WINK, Auburn Professor of Biblical Interpretation at Union Theological Seminary in Manhattan, is well-known and respected for his groundbreaking trilogy on "the powers"—*Naming the Powers: the Language of Power in the New Testament; Unmasking the Powers: The Invisible Forces That Determine Human Existence;* and *Engaging the Powers: Discernment and Resistance in a World of Domination.* He has also written a wonderful book on Bible study called *The Bible in Human Transformation.*

But writing theological books has not made Walter immune to personal faith questions. Like anyone else he has struggled with his faith. Walter's crisis of faith, which culminated on September 11, actually began during the summer of 2000 when Nancy, his beloved daughter-in-law, fell gravely ill and quickly went into a coma. Just before her illness, Nancy's commitment to a spiritual journey had deepened, and she had dreamed that she was in a new, beautifully furnished home. Nancy had felt the dream signaled wonderful new possibilities for her life. At the time no one in her family could imagine that the home in her dream might mean her eternal home. Although lavished with love and prayers for healing, Nancy never emerged from her coma.

When Nancy died on July 5, 2000, Walter and his wife felt utterly devastated and robbed of a daughter. "Her death was our personal 9/11," he says. He remembers feeling like the rabbis in a concentration camp who staged a trial against God. After much discussion, they found God guilty as charged—God had done nothing to stop the slaughter of the Jews. Even with that verdict hanging in the air, the rabbis nevertheless immediately began their evening prayers.

Unlike the rabbis, Walter stopped praying for four or five months after Nancy's death. Finally he resumed praying because, as he says, "people need prayer," and he couldn't help but pray, especially after the trauma of the terrorist attack. "Although Hiroshima and Nagasaki were worse, September 11 was the most horrifying thing most of us have ever seen," Walter says. "In a way, we were there."

As the smoke covered the sky that day, so was the face of God obscured for many. However, Walter believes that even though hidden, God was surely present on September 11, just as God was present but hidden during the time of Nancy's dying. Hidden or visible, God draws "the rabbis" to prayer.

Months later, Walter still struggles with how to respond as a person of faith in this new world. Obviously terrorism must be stopped, yet he strongly questions the wisdom of abandoning nonviolence to destroy the terrorist network, for it means that many innocent people will get hurt or die in the process. What are the guidelines in a world in which thousands of militants are willing to commit suicide, made radical partly by our own national policies and lifestyle?

Of one thing Walter is sure: Satan, as the spirit of what he calls "the Domination System," blinds us to our own evil impulses and deeds. He sees the Domination System at work in conversations that label the United States as "good" and "innocent" and the other side as "evil" or "the axis of evil." He sees it in the blanket distrust of Muslims and in the easy slide into rhetoric of sweet revenge.

What captures Walter's heart these days is what he calls the "acid test": Jesus' teachings on loving enemies as a way to overcome domination. As Walter says in *Engaging the Powers,* "There is, in fact, no other way to God for our time but through the enemy, for loving the enemy has become the key both to human survival in the nuclear age and to personal transformation."[1]

PRAYER SUGGESTION

Let Walter Wink's acid test of loving your enemies challenge you. Whom do you need to learn to love? Perhaps someone who betrayed or abandoned you? someone who slandered or cheated you? a cruel parent or spouse? the terrorists? What hinders you from loving wholeheartedly? If you are not sure, try looking at the suggestions on pages 152–53 for working with anger.

After writing your response in your journal, think about whether you can willingly ask God to help you love your enemies and remove whatever obstacles are in the way. If you are not yet ready, tell God that as well.

If you are ready, with God's help, to risk loving someone who has hurt you personally, discern how best to contact that person and seek reconciliation. If the person is dead or refuses to talk to you, imagine him or her sitting near you. Speak aloud your words of love and forgiveness as you ask God to create love for this person in you. How do you imagine the person responds? How do you respond? Remember that God can empower you to love your enemies even if they don't love you in return.

Record your experience in your journal.

1. Walter Wink, *Engaging the Powers: Discernment and Resistance in a World of Domination* (Minneapolis, Minn.: Fortress Press, 1992), 263.

Joy

ANNE MIMI SAMMIS is an internationally recognized artist who lives and works in Narragansett, Rhode Island. Her soaring, dancing bronze sculptures, which have been exhibited at the United Nations and The Hague, are infused with hope and pure joy. (See the photos throughout this book for samples of Mimi's work.) Her sculptures are partly a prayer of thanksgiving for her own healing, for Mimi's creations emerge out of both her personal healing journey and her vibrant faith in God.

A devout Episcopalian, Mimi often prays as she walks along the ocean in front of her house. For months after the attacks of September 11, Mimi felt a new intensity of joy in the presence of Christ. In January 2002 her sense of Jesus' presence deepened even more. "It's as if his energy is passing though me. I feel him as love, light, creativity, hope, faith, joy, wisdom, power, joy! It's as if he speaks into my being, 'I am the way, and the truth, and the life.'" In response, Mimi finds herself praying this prayer:

> Lord, make me an instrument of thy peace;
> where there is hatred, let me sow love;
> where there is injury, pardon;
> where there is doubt, faith;

where there is despair, hope;
where there is darkness, light;
and where there is sadness, joy.

O Divine Master,
grant that I may not so much seek
to be consoled as to console;
to be understood, as to understand;
to be loved, as to love;
for it is in giving that we receive,
it is in pardoning that we are pardoned,
and it is in dying that we are born to eternal life.
  —attributed to Saint Francis of Assisi; actual
    origin unknown

PRAYER SUGGESTION

How do you react to Mimi's gift of the joy of Christ? Inspired and moved? Envious? Doubtful? Angry? Or some other way? Tell Christ how you feel and open yourself to his response to you. Record what happens in your journal.

Remember that it is possible to feel joy even when your world has come apart. Joy is not the same as happiness; it is not reserved only for times when everything is going well. Joy is knowing that you are rooted in Christ, no matter what.

You can't create joy in yourself, but you can pray for it. If you feel ready, pray daily for the gift of joy; and, as best you can, make a space inside yourself for joy to grow. Let God plant and tend the seeds over time. In the following weeks and months, record with thanksgiving any glimmers of joy in your journal.

☞ Try praying the prayer on pages 179–80 slowly, as if it were your own. What parts of the prayer are difficult for you to pray with honesty? What part of this prayer do you need to omit for now? Write about your experience in your journal.

AFTERWORD

Holding Hands with Crucifixion and Resurrection

⁓

As you heal more and more deeply, God invites you to be present to both crucifixion and resurrection. You must not lose sight of either one, for the whole truth sets you free. Again and again God calls you to embrace both the reality of profound suffering and tragedy and the magnificent truth that in Christ death is swallowed up in victory.

When you are passionately willing to hold hands with both suffering and joy, entering into the depth of crucifixion and resurrection, you may discover a new and astonishing truth: There is a place of contemplative rest and profound healing between the two. When crucifixion and resurrection mingle in a human heart, it is a sign of God making all things new. Resting here, you do not need to hold onto awareness; rather it holds onto you. You do not need to form words of explanation about what is happening—indeed you cannot—but you can allow God to penetrate your being with mystery. In this holy place, you begin to see the whole truth, both tragedy and its transformation. Suffering, seen through the lens of resurrection, is a birthing place of faith; in this crucible, suffering often turns into gift. Here you discover the peace that passes all understanding. Here you know that God provides healing, not just for your individual comfort, as important as that is, but that God also reaches out in love to care for all of humanity. From here you are sent, imperfect as you are, to become intoxicated with love for the world, reflecting the Christ you follow. And you will return to this place—between cross and resurrection—again and again to be healed.

About the Author

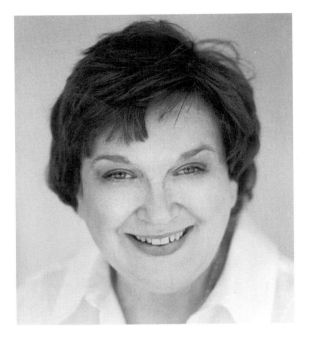

TILDA NORBERG, a United Methodist minister and a Gestalt psychotherapist, is the founder of Gestalt Pastoral Care. This holistic form of pastoral counseling combines Gestalt psychotherapy, healing prayer, and spiritual companioning. In addition to her private psychotherapy practice, Norberg leads workshops and retreats for a variety of groups. For more information about her work, see the author's Web site at www.gestaltpastoralcare.com.

In 1984 Norberg established a two-year training program in Gestalt Pastoral Care for clergy and therapists. As a psychotherapist, she has worked extensively with trauma survivors. She is the author of *Threadbear: A Story of Christian Healing for Adult Survivors of Sexual Abuse* and coauthor (with Robert Webber) of *Stretch Out Your Hand: Exploring Healing Prayer.*

Norberg is a graduate of Union Theological Seminary in New York City, The Gestalt Institute of Canada, and the Lomi School in San Francisco. She is married to Reverend George McClain, and they have two grown children: Shana Norberg-McClain and Noah Norberg-McClain.

About the Artist

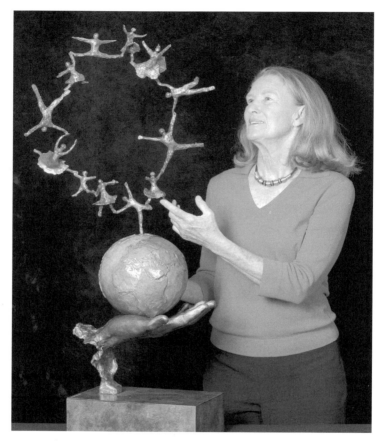

It is my hope that my sculpture touches, inspires, and validates the peace that is within each one of us. I feel strongly that love is the healer of everything. When people come into contact with art, if love and joy are represented, the response and interaction with it can raise the consciousness of the world.

—Anne Mimi Sammis

ANNE MIMI SAMMIS, a renowned artist and sculptor, created the sculptures featured in this book. Sammis's works are represented in more than three hundred public and private collections around the world. They have been exhibited at the United Nations, The Hague (Netherlands), and at Lambeth Palace in London.

Sammis's sculptures reflect her passion for love and peace. She says, "These pieces are about love of self, love of others, love of God. Any interaction of love between human beings touches me, and I am moved to create."

Educated at Yale and the Rhode Island School of Design, Sammis currently lives and works in Narrangansett, Rhode Island and San Miguel de Allende, Mexico.

For more information, see the artist's Web site at www.mimisammis.com.

Don't Miss These Titles on Healing

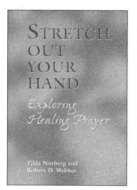

Stretch Out Your Hand
Exploring Healing Prayer
by Tilda Norberg and Robert D. Webber

In *Stretch Out Your Hand,* Tilda Norberg and Robert Webber write candidly about their growing faith in God's desire to bring wholeness. They convey insights into healing prayer through shared spiritual and pastoral wisdom, biblical reflection, and stories from their ministries. The authors address questions that many people ask, such as: Why doesn't everyone who prays get healed? What is the role of faith in healing?

Norberg and Webber open us to the basic truth that healing prayer is more than getting well from an illness; it is part of a beautiful and dynamic process that leads to the wholeness that God wills for us.

ISBN 0-8358-0872-6 • Paperback • 144 pages

To order any of the books mentioned here, visit our online bookstore at www.upperroom.org or call 1-800-972-0433.

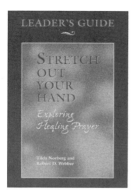

Stretch Out Your Hand
Leader's Guide
by Tilda Norberg and
Robert D. Webber

This study guide, intended to assist those studying the book *Stretch Out Your Hand*, offers guidance for a six-week study.

ISBN 0-8358-0871-8 • Paperback • 48 pages

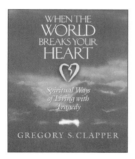

When the World Breaks Your Heart
Spiritual Ways of Living with Tragedy
by Gregory S. Clapper

When United Airlines Flight 232 crashed in 1989, 113 people died and 183 people survived. In this book Gregory S. Clapper, a National Guard chaplain, renders a firsthand account of this tragic event and its aftermath. The author provides six spiritual ways to live with tragedies and includes reflection questions with each chapter to help readers live faithfully in the midst of calamity.

ISBN 0-8358-0842-4 • Paperback • 112 pages

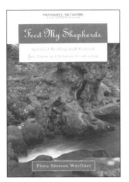

Feed My Shepherds
**Spiritual Healing and Renewal
for Those in Christian Leadership**
by Flora Slosson Wuellner

In *Feed My Shepherds,* Flora Wuellner writes, "While all Christians need nurture and sustenance, the active Christian leader who daily encounters spiritual and emotional stress has special, urgent needs."

An ordained minister in the United Church of Christ, Wuellner knows well that the vocation of Christian leadership can be overwhelmingly demanding, potentially wounding, and stressful. Writing from both her personal experience and her many years as a spiritual counselor and retreat leader, she affirms the urgency of this deep need within Christian leaders to be bonded through Christ to the heart of God. She offers reflection questions and guided meditations to draw the reader into this sustaining relationship.

ISBN 0-8358-0845-9 • Hardcover • 192 pages

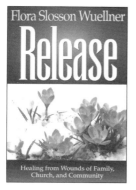

Release
Healing from Wounds of Family, Church, and Community
by Flora Slosson Wuellner

Release focuses on wounds and burdens that did not begin with us but rather were inherited from family or communal generational pain or from unhealed people and communities around us. This book addresses the following questions: What are the signs and symptoms of inherited or internalized suffering? What are the avenues, the ways of release and healing from these burdens? How can we pray for communities—families, churches, workplaces, nations, ethnic groups—that have unhealed wounds and burdens?

The book offers practical help to the reader through Christ-centered reflection, prayer, and biblically based meditations.

ISBN 0-8358-0775 • Paperback • 112 pages